Transitions to Professional Nursing Practice

2nd Edition

by Jamie Murphy, RN, PhD

Associate Professor

SUNY Delhi
School of Nursing
Delhi, New York

SUNY OER SERVICES

2020

Published by SUNY OER Services

SUNY Office of Library and Information Services
10 N Pearl St
Albany, NY 12207

Image credits: Pixabay

Cover design by Jamie Murphy. Cover image by Dave Hoefler on Unsplash located at https://unsplash.com/photos/PEkfSAxeplg

Proper attribution for *Transitions to Professional Nursing Practice*: Transitions to Professional Nursing Practice. Authored by: Jamie Murphy. Provided by: SUNY Delhi. Located at: https://courses.lumenlearning.com/suny-delhi-professionalnursing. License: CC BY: Attribution

ISBN: 978-1-64176-090-4

Contents

Introduction

This text provides a pivotal learning experience for students transitioning from an associate degree education to a baccalaureate degree. Content includes a broad overview of the nursing profession, the role of accrediting and professional organizations with a strong focus on the American Nurses Association's foundational documents. The competencies of the Standards of Professional Practice and the *Code of Ethics* are weaved throughout the text.

Topics covered in this text include professional nursing practice, baccalaureate education, healthcare in the 21st century, autonomy and accountability, nursing philosophy, professional development, communication, interprofessional collaboration, critical thinking, introduction to evidence-based practice, and nursing leadership and theory.

CHAPTER 1

Professional Nursing Practice

Nursing practice has evolved over the centuries, beginning with Florence Nightingale in the 19th century conducting her own research on caring for soldiers in the Crimean War, to contemporary nursing practice in the 21st century where healthcare delivery has become complex, requiring a highly educated nursing workforce to meet the needs of a diverse, aging population.

This opening chapter on professional nursing practice begins with the definition of nursing. The American Nurses Association (ANA, 2015c) defines the concept of nursing:

> Nursing is the protection, promotion, and optimization of health and abilities, prevention of illness and injury, facilitation of healing, alleviation of suffering through the diagnosis and treatment of human response, and advocacy in the care of individuals, families, groups, communities, and populations (p. 1)

Nursing: An Art and a Science

Nursing has been referred to as an art and a science since the early 20th century when nurse licensure laws were first enacted. The concepts art and science are considered the defining characteristics of nursing, thus helping nurses understand and explain the nature of nursing practice (Peplau, 1988).

Art of Nursing

In the mid-nineteenth century, the art of nursing was characterized as mothering and homemaking. A century later, the art of nursing was referred to as "nursing arts", characterized as bathing, bedmaking, positioning patients, comforting techniques, and hospital housekeeping (. , 1981).

Peplau (1988) categorizes the art of nursing as ". . . enabling, empowering, or transforming art. It's aim, among other goals, is to produce favorable changes within clients through nursing services" (p. 9). People are changed on a personal level as a result of the acts provided by nurses (Peplau, 1988). Creating trusting relationships with patients, and others, comes from the art of nursing, it gives nurses the opportunity to speak freely and honestly, to counsel and share their thoughts, knowledge, and feelings in a caring, genuine way.

Pagana (1987) suggests ". . . nurses are major keepers of the morality, goodness, honesty, ethics of client care, [often referred to as] a patient advocate" (p. 9). Expressions associated with the art of nursing includes "individualized care", "uniqueness of the patient", and "the patient as a person" (Peplau, 1988, p. 9). The art of nursing relies on nurses using common sense, reflection of client experiences, and personal observation (Peplau, 1988).

Today, the ANA (2015c) describes the art of nursing as the act of caring and respect for human dignity. Approaching care in a compassionate way brings about competent care. Embracing spirituality, healing, empathy, mutual respect and compassion promotes health and healing. Nurses express art through helping, listening, mentoring, coaching, touching, intuition, cultural competence, tolerance, acceptance, and nurturing.

Many of the attributes of the art of nursing are an inherent part of nursing practice, such as respect for human dignity and compassion. Though some nurses may need to learn some of these attributes through observation of others, such as touching and nurturing. Consider how the art of nursing can be taught in nursing school or learned/strengthened throughout one's career.

A Caring Profession

Nursing is a caring profession, and those who enter the profession often do so for altruistic reasons. People are attracted to the profession because of their desire to help those in need, those who are vulnerable. Gormley (1996) writes "Altruism represents an amalgamation of intrinsic and extrinsic factors which either permit or coerce individuals to take responsibility for or care for another and to sacrifice things dearly held" (p. 581). When caring originates from a group of altruistic individuals, called collective altruism, such as a hospital unit, the generalized concern results in the success of the group's goals and desires (Gormley, 1996).

Nursing theorists have studied the nature of caring and how it impacts both the patient and the nurse. Watson (1988) explains how nurses assist patients to find meaning in their illness by protecting them and preserving human dignity through caring moments. These caring moments lead patients to self-discovery and self-knowledge. For example, the act of holding a patient's hand the night before surgery or listening to a grieving patient's sorrow become long-lasting memories for both the patient and the nurse.

Science of Nursing

Up until the 1940s, the science of nursing was considered knowledge gleaned from science courses during nursing education. By the 1970s, the science of nursing was referred to as systematized knowledge and became a more significant component in nursing education (Peplau, 1988).

As time passed, nurses wanted to further the professionalization of nursing practice. In order for nursing to be considered a profession, science needed to become a more significant component of practice (Peplau, 1988). According to the ANA (1980), a profession must include the use of scientific knowledge to understand and treat phenomena. Through use of scientific inquiry, nurses use theory to investigate and explain phenomenon, determine interventions, and design a plan of care (ANA, 1980). The science of nursing explained the patterns and problems of human beings as a group (Peplau, 1988).

Today, a chief component of nursing practice includes application of evidence-based practice and research in the clinical setting, and scientific investigation. Nurses are actively involved in scientific research at academic institutions as well as the federal level. The National Institute of Nursing Research (NINR, n.d.) is a federally funded nursing research program with a focus on improving population health through scientific research in behavioral and biological sciences. Additional information on NINRs research programs can be found at the National Institute of Nursing Research website.

As a scientific discipline, nursing draws on knowledge from scientific research, nursing theory, the relationship between patients, nurses, and the environment within the context of health, theories from science, humanities, and other related disciplines.

Foundational Documents of Professional Nursing

The ANA has developed three foundational documents for registered nurses, listed below. These documents were written for all registered nurses and are used to inform their thinking and decision-making in nursing practice settings.

- *Code of Ethics for Nurses with Interpretive Statements*
- *Nursing: Scope and Standards of Practice.*
- *Nursing's Social Policy Statement: The Essence of the Profession*

Code of Ethics for Nurses with Interpretive Statements

The **Code of Ethics** is an expression of the values, duties, and commitments of registered nurses. The first **Code of Ethics** was written in 1893 in the form of a pledge similar to the Hippocratic Oath and is now a living document that continually evolves in accordance with the changing social context of nursing (ANA, 2015a).

Provision 1	**Affirming health through relationships of dignity and respect** • 1.1 Respect for human dignity • 1.2 Relationships with patients • 1.3 The nature of health • 1.4 The right to self-determination • 1.5 Relationships with colleagues and others (ANA, 2015a, pp1-18)
Provision 2	**The patient as nursing's foundational commitment** • 2.1 Primacy of the patient's interests • 2.2 Conflict of interest for nurses • 2.3 Collaboration • 2.4 Professional boundaries (ANA, 2015a, pp. 25-35)
Provision 3	**Advocacy's geography** • 3.1 Protection of the rights of privacy and confidentiality • 3.2 Protection of human participants in research • 3.3 Performance standards and review mechanisms • 3.4 Professional responsibility in promoting a culture of safety • 3.5 Protection of patient health and safety by action on questionable practice • 3.6 Patient protection and impaired practice (ANA, 2015a, pp. 41-53)
Provision 4	**The expectations of expertise** • 4.1 Authority, accountability, and responsibility • 4.2 Accountability for nursing judgments, decisions, and actions • 4.3 Responsibility for nursing judgments, decisions, and actions • 4.4 Assignment and delegation of nursing activities or tasks (ANA, 2015a, pp. 59-68)
Provision 5	**The nurse as person of dignity and worth** • 5.1 Duties to self and others • 5.2 Promotion of personal health, safety, and well-being • 5.3 Preservation of wholeness of character • 5.4 Preservation of integrity • 5.5 Maintenance of competence and continuation of professional growth • 5.6 Continuation of personal growth (ANA, 2015a, pp. 73-90)
Provision 6	**The moral milieu of nursing practice** • 6.1 The environment and moral virtue • 6.2 The environment and ethical obligation • 6.3 Responsibility for the healthcare environment (ANA, 2015a, pp. 95-105)
Provision 7	**Diverse contributions to the profession** • 7.1 Contributions through research and scholarly inquiry • 7.2 Contributions through developing, maintaining, and implementing professional practice standards • 7.3 Contributions through nursing and health policy development (ANA, 2015a, pp. 113-122)
Provision 8	**Collaboration to reach for greater ends** • 8.2 Health is a universal right • 8.3 Collaboration for health, human rights, and health diplomacy • 8.4 Obligation to advance health and human rights and reduce disparities • 8.5 Collaboration for human rights in complex, extreme, or extraordinary practice settings (ANA, 2015a, pp. 129-140)
Provision 9	**Social justice: Reaching out to a world in need of nursing** • 9.1 Articulation and assertion of values • 9.2 Integrity of the profession • 9.3 Integrating social justice • 9.4 Social justice in nursing and health policy (ANA, 2015a, pp. 151-160)

Nursing: Scope and Standards of Practice

The ANA (2015c) *Nursing: Scope and Standards of Practice* contains the Scope of Nursing Practice and the Standards of Professional Nursing Practice. The latter is comprised of the Standards of Practice (standards 1-6) and the Standards of Professional Performance (standards 7-17).

Scope of Nursing Practice

The scope describes the activities performed by the nurse as the *who, what, where, when, why,* and *how* nursing is practiced (ANA, 2015c). Responses to these questions are answered "to provide a complete picture of the dynamic and complex practice of nursing" (ANA, 2015c, p. 2). The following describes how each of these questions are answered:

- **Who:** the registered nurse
- **What:** this is the definition of nursing, as listed above.
- **Where:** any place there is a need for care, advocacy, or knowledge
- **When:** anytime there is a need for nursing knowledge, wisdom, leadership, caring
- **Why:** nurses need to maintain the social contract with society, adapting care based on the changing needs of the society
- **How:** the method and manner to which nurses practice professionally (ANA, 2015c, p. 2)

Standards of Practice

The Standards of Practice describe a competent level of nursing care expected of all registered nurses, regardless of their role, specialty, or position. The depth and breadth of how nurses employ these practices are dependent upon level of education, self-development, experience, role, setting, and patient population being served (ANA, 2015b). These Standards are often referred to as the nursing process or the acronym *ADPIE* (assessment, diagnosis, planning, implementation and evaluation). Registered nurses are expected to demonstrate critical thinking throughout all actions taken during each standard, which forms the foundation for decision-making (ANA, 2015c). See Table 1 for the Standards of Practice.

Table 1 lists the 6 Standards of Practice

Table 1: Standards of Practice

Standard 1: Assessment	The registered nurse collects pertinent data and information relative to the healthcare consumer's health or the situation.
Standard 2: Diagnosis	The registered nurse analyzes the assessment data to determine actual or potential diagnoses, problems, and issues.
Standard 3: Outcomes Identification	The registered nurse identifies expected outcomes for a plan individualized to the healthcare consumer or the situation.
Standard 4: Planning	The registered nurse develops a plan that prescribes strategies to attain expected, measurable outcomes.
Standard 5: Implementation	The registered nurse implements the identified plan
Standard 5A: Coordination of Care	The registered nurse coordinates care delivery.
Standard 5B: Health Teaching and Health Promotion	The registered nurse employs strategies to promote health and a safe environment.
Standard 6: Evaluation	The registered nurse evaluates progress toward attainment of goals and outcomes.
	(ANA, 2015c, pp. 56-66)

Standards of Professional Performance

The Standards of Professional Performance describes competent behaviors of the professional registered nurse, depending on role, position, and level of education. Some standards may or may not be applicable to patient care. Registered nurses are expected to engage in professional activities related to their role, such as leadership, formal or informal, based upon level of education. Registered nurses are held accountable to themselves, the healthcare consumer, peers, employer, and society as they carry out the competencies of each standard (ANA, 2010). See Table 2 for the Standards of Professional Performance.

Table 2 lists the Standards of Professional Performance

Table 2: Standards of Professional Performance

Standard 7: Ethics	The registered nurse practices ethically.
Standard 8: Culturally Congruent Practice	The registered nurse practices in a manner that is congruent with cultural diversity and inclusion principles.
Standard 9: Communication	The registered nurse communicates effectively in all areas of practice.
Standard 10: Collaboration	The registered nurse collaborates with the healthcare consumer and other key stakeholders in the conduct of nursing practice.
Standard 11: Leadership	The registered nurse leads within the professional practice setting and the profession.
Standard 12: Education	The registered nurse seeks knowledge and competence that reflects current nursing practice and promotes futuristic thinking.
Standard 13: Evidence-Based Practice and Research	The registered nurse integrates evidence and research findings into practice.
Standard 14: Quality of Practice	The registered nurse contributes to quality nursing practice.
Standard 15: Professional Practice Evaluation	The registered nurse evaluates one's own and others' nursing practice.
Standard 16: Resource Utilization	The registered nurse utilizes appropriate resources to plan, provide, and sustain evidence-based nursing services that are safe, effective, and fiscally responsible.
Standard 17: Environmental Health	The registered nurse practice in an environmentally safe and healthy manner.

(ANA, 2015c, pp. 67-84)

Nursing's Social Policy Statement: The Essence of the Profession

Nursing's social policy statement describes the value of the nursing profession within society, defines the concept of nursing, reviews the standards of practice, and regulation of nursing practice. The nursing practice is inherently connected to society, thus requiring a social contract between society and the profession (ANA, 2015b).

Nursing's core values and ethics serve as a social contract to society, which provides a foundation for the health of society. Through licensure, affirmation, and legislation, society validates the need for and trust in nursing profession. The nursing profession meets society's need to obtain healthcare, regardless of cultural, social, or economic standing (ANA, 2015b).

Since 2001, the Gallup poll found Americans ranked nurses as the most trustworthy, with the highest ethical standards compared to 21 other professions (Reinhart, 2020). The nursing profession is trusted by society to provide quality, ethical care. Society gives permission to the profession of nursing to work autonomously to meet the needs of society as a whole. In return, the nursing profession is expected to provide healthcare in a responsible manner while maintaining the public's trust (Donabedian, 1976).

Accrediting and Professional Organizations

There are several important organizations and documents that have significant impact on practice, education, and professional growth. Below is a list of organizations and research reports that have are foundational to implementing practices that ensure high standards of care.

American Nurses Association

The American Nurses Association (ANA, n.d.-a) was founded in 1896 with the goal of advancing the nursing profession and improving the quality of care for all. Since its inception well over a century ago, membership is widespread throughout all 50 states and U.S. territories, and known as the "strongest voice of the profession". The ANA advances the profession through the development many foundational documents, white papers, position statements, initiatives, among others:

- Standards of Practice and Performance for nursing including practice-focused standards for 25 nursing specialties
- Code of Ethics
- Social Policy Statement
- Advocacy efforts with health policy and safe working environments
- Research and funding opportunities
- Self-care for nurses
- Lobbying Congress

The ANA (n.d.-a) fights for what nurses need, what they believe in, and supports nurses to lead change in this ever-evolving healthcare environment. The ANA empowers nurses in the hopes of making positive changes in healthcare and fighting for what their patients need. Below are some of the efforts the ANA continues to work towards:

- Expanded roles for RNs and Advanced Practice Registered Nurses (APRN)
- Federal funding for nursing education and training
- Improvement of the healthcare environment
- Medicare reform
- Safe staffing
- Workplace violence
- Whistleblowing protection

The ANA (n.d.-b) has developed the following organizational platforms focused on nursing excellence:

- Magnet Recognition Program
- Pathway to Excellence
- American Nurses Credentialing Center
- ANA Enterprise
- American Nurses Foundation
- ANCC Accreditation
- ANA Certifications

For more information about ANA's programs and services, visit the ANA website.

National League for Nursing

The National League for Nursing (NLN, 2020) was founded in 1893 as the as the American Society of Superintendents of Training Schools for Nurses, the first U.S. professional nursing organization. The NLN is considered the premier organization for nursing education. Membership includes individual faculty members and leaders in nursing education including healthcare organizations and agencies. The organization offers its 40,000 individual members and 1200 institutional members a wide array of services and opportunities:

- Professional development
- Networking
- Research and grant opportunities
- Testing services
- Recognition programs
- Certification for nurse educators
- Advocacy and public policy initiatives.
- Commission for Nursing Education Accreditation (CNEA) activities for associate, diploma, baccalaureate, and post-graduate degree nursing programs.

For more information about the NLN, visit the NLN website.

American Association of Colleges of Nursing

The American Association of Colleges of Nursing (AACN, 2020b) was founded in 1969 as the voice of academic nursing education. Some of the major activities of the AACN include establishment of quality standards for nursing education, assist nursing schools on how to be implement quality standards, and promote public support of nursing education, research, and practice. Membership includes 814 schools of nursing that offer baccalaureate, graduate, and post-graduate programs, 45,000 individual members, with 513,000 students. AACN (2020b) offers the following programs, foundational documents, and initiatives:

- *Essentials of Baccalaureate Education for Professional Nursing Practice.* To view the Essentials document, visit the AACN website.
- *Position Statement: The Baccalaureate Degree in Nursing as Minimal Preparation for Professional Practice.* To view the *Position Statement,* visit the AACN website.
- Curriculum standards: includes the *Essentials* documents, which outlines the competencies for graduates of baccalaureate, master's, and Doctor of Nursing Practice (DNP) degrees
- Conferences and webinars
- Grant funding
- Policy and Advocacy
- Commission on Collegiate Nursing Education (CCNE) Accreditation activities for baccalaureate, graduate, and residency programs in nursing
- Certifications
- Journals, white papers, position statements, faculty tool kits, and more
  For more information about AACN, visit the AACN website.

National Council of State Boards of Nursing

The National Council of State Boards of Nursing (NCSBN, 2020b) was founded in 1978 as an independent, not-for-profit organization. The NCSBN's core goal is focused on ensuring safe patient care and protecting the public through implementation of unbiased regulation (NCSBN, 2020c). NCSBN membership consists of the following boards of nursing (BON):

- 50 U.S. states, including District of Columbia
- Four U.S. territories: American Samoa, Guam, Northern Mariana Islands, and the Virgin Islands
- Three states have two BONs; one for RNs and one for LPNs: California, Louisiana, and West Virginia
- Nebraska has the BON for RNs and the BON for advanced practice nurses (NCSBN, 2020a)

The NCSBN (2020b) is responsible for the following activities:

- Regulation of over 4.8 million nurses
- Developed the National Council Licensure Examination (NCLEX-RN and NCLEX-PN)
- Collaborative research
- Position papers
- Nursing disciplinary database
- Verification of nursing licensure
- Practice privileges
- Nurse Practice Act designed and published (*see Accountability chapter for more information*)
- Gathers national data on RNs, LPNs
- Publishes the *Journal of Nursing Regulation*

For more information about NCSBN, visit the NCSBN website.

National Academy of Sciences and the Health and Medicine Division

The Health and Medicine Division (HMD) (formerly the Institute of Medicine (IOM)) is part of the National Academies of Sciences, Engineering, and Medicine (NAS). The organization has been in operation since 1863. The NAS conducts research by request from federal agencies, independent organizations, or by Congressional mandate. The NAS is responsible for conducting objective research that is used to advise and inform public policy in relation to science, technology, and medicine. The overarching goal of HMD is to inform those working in both the government and the private sectors on how to make healthcare decisions by providing reliable, objective, and informative research findings (NAS, 2020).

The NAS conducts research on a variety of healthcare topics, including aging, health literacy, obesity, cancer, social determinants of health, among others. For more information about NAS research, visit the NAS website.

Previous to the naming of the NAS organization, the IOM published landmark reports on *The Future of Nursing* (listed below) which explore nursing roles, responsibilities, standards of practice, education, among other topics. These reports were conducted to meet the needs of a diverse, aging, and complex healthcare environment.

- To view the report on the *Future of Nursing: Leading Change, Advancing Health,* download the PDF file in week 1.

For more information about NAS, visit the NAS website.

Characteristics of a Profession

Brown (1992) explains the origins of the concept *profession* from 1675. The concept was first used in secular society with the following definition: "... to define, organize, and publicize their own particular expertise and cultural authority (p. 18)". Many occupations today have similarities with this definition. Consider the professions of nursing, lawyers, and accountants requiring a particular expertise. They are all organized entities, publicized to those who are in need of such expertise, and they subscribe to a particular culture or way of being.

Today, scholars have defined particular characteristics of a profession in order to differentiate from an occupation. Buhai (2012) lists the following characteristics of a profession:

- specialized training/education
- autonomy of practice
- ethical practice
- expert knowledge
- trust
- self-regulation
- continuing education
- service to society

Nursing has been referred to as a profession for many years, meeting all of the above characteristics, though its status as a profession has been debated. One of the characteristics of a profession under debate is the educational requirement, entry level to practice. Nursing offers multiple pathways to practice, including diploma, associate, and baccalaureate. Each program of study varies widely with depth and breadth of nursing content, though each graduate takes the same licensure exam (Krugman & Goode, 2018).

By the early 21st century, disciplines within the healthcare field have increased minimum preparation for practice to higher levels of education, including physical therapy (master's degree or doctorate) and pharmacy (doctorate) (Krugman & Goode, 2018). Since nursing does not have a clear pathway to practice (Blais & Hayes, 2011; Krugman & Goode, 2018) it has been argued that nursing has still not met the educational requirement of a profession (Joel & Kelly, 2002). Until the entry to practice issue is resolved, some may not consider nursing as a true profession.

Characteristics of Professional Nursing Practice

The ANA (2015c) lists five core tenets of nursing practice, all of which are weaved throughout the standards of practice and professional performance:

1. Caring and health are central to the practice of the registered nurse

Professional nursing promotes healing and health in a way that builds a relationship between nurse and patient (Watson, 2012).

2. Nursing practice is individualized

Respect for human dignity and diversity is at the core of identifying and meeting the unique needs of the healthcare consumer or situation (ANA, 2015c, p. 8).

3. Registered nurses use the nursing process to plan and provide individualized care for healthcare consumers

Nurses apply the six standards of practice during encounters with the healthcare consumer, groups, or populations. The use of theory and evidence-based knowledge is used to collaborate with the healthcare consumer [or others] to achieve the best outcomes (ANA, 2015c, p. 8).

4. Nurses coordinate care by establishing partnerships

Partnerships with persons, families, groups, support systems, and other stakeholders should be established using multiple forms of communication. Share goal-setting should include delivery of safe, quality care (ANA, 2015c, p. 8).

5. A strong link exists between the professional work environment and the registered nurse's ability to provide quality health care and achieve optimal outcomes

Nurses have an ethical obligation to create healthy practice environments that are conducive to provision of quality healthcare (ANA, 2015c, p. 9)

See chapter 4, Leadership in Nursing, for more information about healthy working environments

Competencies for Professional Nursing Practice

The ANA (2014) published a Position Statement on Professional Role Competence for all registered nurses. The following summarizes the main points of the Position Statement, outlining the expectations of society, nurses, the profession, and employers:

- The public has a right to expect all nurses demonstrate competence in their role throughout their career
- Nurses are responsible and accountable for maintaining role competence
- The nursing profession and regulatory agencies verify the processes for measuring competence is appropriate, and they meet the minimum standards to protect the general public
- Employers are responsible and accountable for providing a safe working environment conducive to competent practice

To view the Position Statement on Professional Role Competence, visit the ANA website

Massachusetts Department of Higher Education Nursing (2016) created the Nurse of the Future competencies for professional nursing practice:

- **Patient-Centered Care**

  Provision of "holistic care that recognizes an individual's preferences, values, and needs and respects the patient or designee as a full partner in providing compassionate, coordinated, age and culturally appropriate, safe and effective care" (p. 10)

- **Professionalism**

  "Accountability for the delivery of standard-based nursing care that is consistent with moral, altruistic, legal, ethical, regulatory, and humanistic principles" (p. 14)

- **Leadership**

  "Influence the behavior of individuals or groups of individuals within their environment in a way that will facilitate the establishment and acquisition/achievement of shared goals" (p. 18)\

  see Chapter 4 for more information on nursing leadership

- **Informatics and Technology**

  "Use advanced technology and to analyze as well as synthesize information and collaborate in order to make critical decisions that optimize patient outcomes" (p. 26)

- **Evidenced-Based Practice**

  "Identify, evaluate, and use the best current evidence coupled with clinical expertise and consideration of patients' preferences, experience and values to make practice decisions" (p. 47)

  see Chapter 3 for more information on evidence-based practice

- **Systems-Based Practice**

  "Awareness of and responsiveness to the larger context of the health care system, and will demonstrate the ability to effectively call on work unit resources to provide care that is of optimal quality and value" (p. 20)

- **Safety**

  "Minimize risk of harm to patients and providers through both system effectiveness and individual performance" (p. 42)

- **Communication**

  "interact effectively with patients, families, and colleagues, fostering mutual respect and shared decision making, to enhance patient satisfaction and health outcomes" (p. 32)

  see Chapter 3 for more information on communication

- **Teamwork and Collaboration**

  "Function effectively within nursing and interdisciplinary teams, fostering open communication, mutual respect, shared decision making, team learning, and development" (p. 37)

  see Chapter 3 for more information on teamwork and collaboration

- **Quality Improvement**

  "Use data to monitor the outcomes of care processes, and uses improvement methods to design and test changes to continuously improve the quality and safety of health care systems" (p. 45)

Baccalaureate Education

The goal of nursing education is to prepare nurses with comprehensive knowledge and skills to provide safer nursing care in today's complex healthcare environment. Many changes have occurred in the last 25-50 years and will only accelerate as new technologies develop and demographics continue to change. In addition to healthcare shifting from tertiary care (acute hospital-centered) to community-based settings, the patient population is more diverse, older, and requires care for multiple chronic illnesses. More than ever, nurses need to be prepared with the required competencies and knowledge to practice across multiple settings in order to provide safe, quality care. Obtaining a baccalaureate degree can meet the demand for a highly educated nursing workforce.

Patient-centered care is more important than ever in today's healthcare environment. Providing individualized care requires not only communicating and collaborating effectively with the patient, family, and interdisciplinary team, but to also coordinating care with community partnerships, organizations, and other stakeholders within the healthcare system. Nurses must acquire competence as a provider, designer, manager, and coordinator of care. A baccalaureate education prepares nurses to understand the broader context of healthcare, such as reimbursement and accreditation requirements (American Association of Colleges of Nursing [AACN], 2008).

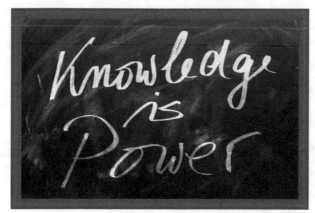

Baccalaureate Education and Impact on Outcomes

The Institute of Medicine (IOM, 2011) studied the overall healthcare environment and the current state of nursing educational readiness. The IOM reported nurses need to attain higher levels of education (minimum of BSN) and a seamless transition to higher levels of education (diploma and associate to BSN) (IOM, 2011). These conclusions are supported by researchers who have studied the competencies of baccalaureate prepared nurses compared to associate degree prepared nurses (See Table 1). An overwhelming number of studies have shown a positive relationship between patient outcomes and care provided by baccalaureate prepared nurses. The following list summarizes the research findings on the impact of a baccalaureate education from Table 1 below:

- Reduced mortality rates
- Stronger leadership skills
- Stronger synthesis and application of knowledge
- Reduced failure to rescue rates
- Reduced rate of decubitus ulcers, postoperative deep vein thrombosis or pulmonary embolism
- Shorter length of stay
- Reduced readmission rates leading to substantial cost savings (AACN, n.d.)

Table 1 below illustrates the results of research studies focused on the level of nursing education and its impact on health outcomes.

Table 1: Evidence on the Impact of Baccalaureate-Level Nursing Education

Reference	Findings
Goode, C.J., Pinkerton, S., McCausland, M.P., Southard, P., Graham, R., & Krsek, C. (2001). Documenting chief nursing officers' preference for BSN-prepared nurses. *Journal of Nursing Administration, 31*(2). 55-59. http://doi.org/10.1097/00005110-200102000-00002	72% of nursing directors identified differences in practice between BSN-prepared RNs and those with an associate degree or hospital diploma; baccalaureate-prepared nurses demonstrated stronger synthesis and application of knowledge and leadership skills.
Aiken, L.H., Clarke, S.P., Cheung, R.B., Sloane, D.M., & Silber, J.H. (2003). Educational levels of hospital nurses and surgical patient mortality. *JAMA, 290*(12), 1617-1623. http://doi.org/10.1001/jama.290.12.1617	Researchers found a clear link between higher levels of nursing education and better patient outcomes. Surgical patients have a "substantial survival advantage" if treated in hospitals with higher proportions of nurses educated at the baccalaureate or higher degree level. In hospitals, a 10% increase in the proportion of nurses holding BSN degrees decreased the risk of patient death and failure to rescue by 5%.
Estabrooks, C.A., Midodzi, W.K., Cummings, G.C., Ricker, K.L., & Giovanetti, P. (2005). The impact of hospital nursing characteristics on 30-day mortality. *Nursing Research, 54*(2), 72-84. http://doi.org/10.1097/00006199-200503000-00002	Baccalaureate-prepared nurses were found have a positive impact on mortality rates following an examination of more than 18,000 patient outcomes at 49 Canadian hospitals.
Tourangeau, A.E, Doran, D.M., McGillis Hall, L., O'Brien Pallas, L., Pringle, D., Tu, J.V., & Cranley, L.A. (2007). Impact of hospital nursing care on 30-day mortality for acute medical patients. *Journal of Advanced Nursing, 57*(1), 32-41. http://doi.org/10.1111/j.1365-2648.2006.04084.x	BSN-prepared nurses had a positive impact on lowering patient mortality rates in this study of 46,993 patients admitted to the hospital with heart attacks, strokes, pneumonia, and blood poisoning. "Hospitals with higher proportions of baccalaureate-prepared nurses tended to have lower 30-day mortality rates. Findings indicated that a 10% increase in the proportion of baccalaureate prepared nurses was associated with 9 fewer deaths for every 1,000 discharged patients."
Aiken, L.H., Clarke, S.P., Sloane, D.M., Lake, E.T. & Cheney, T. (2008). Effects of hospital care environment on patient mortality and nurse outcomes. *Journal of Nursing Administration, 38*(5), 223-229. http://doi.org/10.1097/01.NNA.0000312773.42352.d7	Study confirmed findings from Dr. Aiken's 2003 study, which showed a link between RN education level and patient outcomes. Key finding: a 10% increase in the proportion of BSN nurses on the hospital staff was associated with a 4% decrease in the risk of death.
Friese, C.R, Lake, E.T., Aiken, L.H., Silber, J.H., & Sochalski, J. (2008). Hospital nurse practice environments and outcomes for surgical oncology patients. *Health Services Research, 43*(4), 1145-1163. https://doi.org/10.1111/j.1475-6773.2007.00825.x	Nurses prepared at the baccalaureate-level were linked with lower mortality and failure-to-rescue rates. The authors conclude that "moving to a nurse workforce in which a higher proportion of staff nurses have at least a baccalaureate-level education would result in substantially fewer adverse outcomes for patients."
Kendall-Gallagher, D., Aiken, L., Sloane, D.M., & Cimiotti, J.P. (2011). Nurse specialty certification, inpatient mortality, and failure to rescue. *Journal of Nursing Scholarship, 43*(2), 188-194. https://doi.org/10.1111/j.1547-5069.2011.01391.x	Nurse specialty certification was associated with better patient outcomes, but only when care was provided by nurses with baccalaureate level education. The authors concluded that "no effect of specialization was seen in the absence of baccalaureate education."
Blegen, M.A., Goode, C.J., Park, S.H., Vaughn, T., & Spetz, J. (2013). Baccalaureate education in nursing and patient outcomes. *Journal of Nursing Administration, 43*(2), 89-94. http://doi.org/10.1097/NNA.0b013e31827f2028	Hospitals with a higher percentage of RNs with baccalaureate or higher degrees had lower congestive heart failure mortality, decubitus ulcers, failure to rescue, and postoperative deep vein thrombosis or pulmonary embolism and shorter length of stay.
Kutney-Lee, A., Sloane, D.M., & Aiken, L. (2013). An increase in the number of nurses with baccalaureate degrees is linked to lower rates of post-surgery mortality. *Health Affairs, 32*(3), 579-586. https://doi.org/10.1377/hlthaff.2012.0504	A 10-point increase in the percentage of nurses holding a BSN within a hospital was associated with an average reduction of 2.12 deaths for every 1,000 patients. In patients with complications, there were 7.47 fewer deaths per 1,000 patients.

McHugh, M.D., Kelly, L.A., Smith, H.L., Wu, E.S., Vanak, J.M., & Aiken, L.H. (2013). Lower mortality in magnet hospitals. *Medical Care, 51*(5), 382–388. Doi: 10.1097/ MLR.0b013e3182726cc5	Surgical patients in Magnet hospitals had 14% lower odds of inpatient death within 30 days and 12% lower odds of failure-to-rescue compared with patients cared for in non-Magnet hospitals. The authors conclude that these better outcomes were attributed in large part to investments in highly qualified nurses, including a higher proportion of baccalaureate-prepared nurses.
Aiken, L. H., Sloane, D. M., Bruyneel, L. et al. (2014). Nurse staffing and education and hospital mortality in nine European countries: A retrospective observational study. *Lancet, 383*(9931), 1824-30. http://doi.org/10.1016/ S0140-6736(13)62631-8	An increase in a nurses' workload by one patient increased the likelihood of dying within 30 days of admission by 7% and every 10% increase in bachelor's degree nurses was associated with a decrease in this likelihood by 7%.
Yakusheva, O., Lindrooth, R., & Weiss, M. (2014). Economic evaluation of the 80% baccalaureate nurse workforce recommendation: A patient-level analysis. *Medical Care, 52*(10), 864-869. http://doi.org/10.1097/ MLR.0000000000000189	A 10% increase in the proportion of baccalaureate-prepared nurses on hospital units was associated with lowering patient mortality by 10.9%. Increasing the amount of care provided by BSNs to 80% would result in significantly lower readmission rates and shorter lengths of stay. These outcomes translate into cost savings that would off-set expenses for increasing the number of baccalaureate-prepared nurses in hospitals.
Aiken, L. H., Sloane, D., Griffiths, P., Rafferty, A. M., Bruyneel, L., McHugh, M., Maier, C. B., Moreno-Casbas, T., Ball, J. E., Ausserhoffer, D., & Sermeus, W. (2017). Nursing skill mix in European hospitals: Association with mortality, patient ratings, and quality of care. *BMJ Quality & Safety, 26*(7), 559-568. http://doi.org/10.1136/ bmjqs-2016-005567	A greater proportion of professional nurses at the bedside is associated with better outcomes for patients and nurses. Reducing nursing skill mix by adding assistive personnel without professional nurse qualifications may contribute to preventable deaths, erode care quality, and contribute to nurse shortages.
	(AACN, n.d.)

The Essentials of Baccalaureate Education

As stated in the previous chapter, the AACN (2020b) plays a pivotal role in nursing education and is charged with providing curriculum standards and competencies for baccalaureate, master's, and Doctor of Nursing Practice (DNP) degrees. The following nine competencies for baccalaureate education are outlined in *The Essentials of Baccalaureate Education for Professional Nursing Practice* as follows:

- **Essential I:** Liberal Education for Baccalaureate Generalist Nursing Practice
- **Essential II:** Basic Organizational and Systems Leadership for Quality Care and Patient Safety
- **Essential III:** Scholarship for Evidence Based Practice
- **Essential IV:** Information Management and Application of Patient Care Technology
- **Essential V:** Health Care Policy, Finance, and Regulatory Environments
- **Essential VI:** Interprofessional Communication and Collaboration for Improving Patient Health Outcomes
- **Essential VII:** Clinical Prevention and Population Health
- **Essential VIII:** Professionalism and Professional Values
- **Essential IX:** Baccalaureate Generalist Nursing Practice

The Essentials of Baccalaureate Education for Professional Nursing Practice can be found at the AACN website.

Competencies of Baccalaureate Nurses

Nurses with a baccalaureate degree meet the above competencies, enabling them to secure roles that can transform healthcare to offer safe, quality, and cost-effective care. The following outcomes exemplify some of the characteristics of a professional nurse with a baccalaureate education (AACN, 2008):

- Awareness of vulnerable populations with the knowledge and skill to advocate for such populations
- Identifies best practices and evidence to inform practice to make autonomous clinical judgments
- Develops professional values, and behaviors that are value-based
- Recognizes safety and quality issues
- Awareness of quality improvement action plans, processes, and outcome measures
- Uses the skills of inquiry, critical thinking, and analysis to inform practice

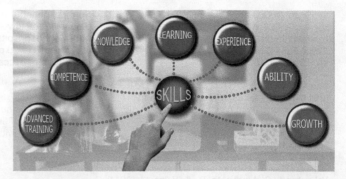

- Through a liberal arts education the nurse has the ability to integrate values, knowledge, and skills to provide care that is safe, high quality, and humanistic
- Practices from a foundation of professional values and standards
- Understands patient (and family, community) values, ensuring a therapeutic relationship that is founded on patient-centered, quality care
- Prepared to identify and manage ethical dilemmas in the workplace
- Able to make and assist others with difficult decision-making within an ethical framework

Academic Progression

The AACN (n.d.) collaborates with academic institutions and community partners to create a highly effective nursing workforce. To that end, AACN has published a position statement on academic progression for registered nurses. In order to meet the complex healthcare demands of the 21st century, and due to the significant impact education has on knowledge and nurse competencies, the AACN proposes the following:

> The American Association of Colleges of Nursing strongly believes that registered nurses (RNs) should be, at minimum, prepared with the Bachelor of Science in Nursing (BSN) or equivalent baccalaureate nursing degree (e.g., BS in Nursing, BA in Nursing) offered at an accredited four-year college or university (AACN, n.d., para. 2).

AACN emphasizes the requirement for lifelong learning as an essential part of nursing practice.

Lifelong learning competencies are weaved throughout the *Baccalaureate Essentials*, which includes outcomes associated with developing professional values, behaviors and sharpened skills of inquiry, critical thinking, and analysis. Lifelong learning is a critical step for progressive learning and personal progress. Jones-Schenk, Leafman, Wallace, and Allen (2017) found that nurses with an associate degree were less likely to have an educational plan than nurses with a bachelor's degrees (Jones-Schenk, Leafman, Wallace, & Allen, 2017).

As a result of the landmark study by the IOM, *The Future of Nursing: Leading Change, Advancing Health*, the nursing profession has strengthened practice through lifelong learning throughout one's career. Mentorship and preceptor programs have been developed to ensure competencies (Pirschel, 2017). Many healthcare organizations have developed residency programs to assist graduate nurses as they acclimate to their new professional roles.

History of the Baccalaureate Degree as the Minimum Preparation

To fully understand the national dialogue about minimum levels of education, it is important to understand how the debate originated and why it's been ongoing on for over 50 years.

In 1960, the American Nurses Association's (ANA, 1965) Committee on Education prepared a proposal asserting a baccalaureate degree should be the basic education for professional nursing practice. After five years, in 1965, the ANA published their first official position statement in *The American Journal of Nursing*. A number of factors were considered before finalizing the position statement, though a number of controversies ensued.

In 1965, Medicare and Medicaid legislation were passed thus ushering in the era of the "Great Society." Older adults and the impoverished were now equally entitled to access to healthcare, and the influx of new patients led to the growth of tertiary care and the need for more nurses (Donley & Flaherty, 2002).

Donley and Flaherty (2002) found three main themes in the writing of the first position statement: 1) autonomy and financial control, 2) nature of nursing practice, and 3) nursing supply. These themes still resonate today, though in slightly different forms.

Autonomy, Finances and the Nature of Nursing Practice

In the American healthcare environment of 1965, nursing education and practice in the hospital setting was controlled by hospitals and their physicians. Over 75% of hospital-based nursing programs centered their curriculum on how to care for acutely ill, hospitalized patients. Since hospitals and physicians had decision-making authority over their nurses, it was a commonly held belief that nursing was merely an occupation (not a profession as it is today) where nurses were handmaidens of physicians. Physician's orders and the care of the old and acutely ill shaped the domain of nursing. The hospital culture was strong, and nurses who were trained in hospital-based programs were ardent supporters of their hospital and physicians. Any change to the status quo of nursing education being centered in the hospital system would take a great deal of persuasion and new ideas (Donley & Flaherty, 2002).

The practice of educating and employing nurses in the hospital setting weakened nursing autonomy due to physicians' premier position in the hospital hierarchy and their authority to make decisions about nursing education (physicians also taught nursing students). After the position statement was published, it was recommended hospitals close down their nursing programs and transition nursing education to colleges and universities. ANA's motivation rested in their belief that nurses were not receiving a comprehensive education and nurses deserved more autonomy over their practice and education (Donley & Flaherty, 2002).

Nursing Supply

The most dramatic response to the publication of the position statement was the growth of associate degree nursing (ADN) programs. See Table 1 below to see the dramatic changes from pre-position statement in 1963 to the data from the National Nursing Workforce Survey in 2017.

Table 2 shares the percent of nurse graduates by program type

Table 2: Percent of Graduates by Program Type

Year	Diploma	ADN	BSN
1963 (Donley & Flaherty, 2002)	75%	5%	20%
2008 (HRSA, 2010)	3%	61%	36%
2013 (Smiley et al., 2018)	13%	32%	40%
2015 (Smiley et al., 2018)	9%	30%	43%
2017 (Smiley et al., 2018)	7%	29%	45%

BSN in 10 Law Passes in New York

A long-standing debate over mandating baccalaureate education in New York ended on December 19, 2017, when Governor Cuomo signed Senate Bill S6768 (BSN in 10). The law states students entering nursing school beginning in 2019 are mandated to obtain a bachelor's degree within 10 years of initial licensure (New York State Senate, 2017). Current registered nurses are not mandated to earn a BSN, though some are returning in order to compete for positions, most often acute care settings. These nurses would be at a competitive disadvantage without a baccalaureate degree since new graduating nurses will be earning their BSN within a relatively short period of time. Mandating a baccalaureate education continues to be hotly debated since the bill has passed for a number of reasons, such as a possible negative impact on the current nursing shortage, financial burden, and more. See the next section for a list of incentives and disincentives for nurses returning to school for a baccalaureate degree.

Proponents of the law include a number of prominent organizations, including:

- Magnet hospitals
- National Advisory Council on Nurse Education and Practice
- U. S. Military (Army, Navy and Air Force)
- Veteran's Administration
- Minority nurse organizations (such as National Black Nurses Association, Hispanic Association of Colleges and Universities)

These organizations acknowledge the value baccalaureate prepared nurses bring to the profession. They also advocate for increasing baccalaureate prepared nurses in all clinical settings (AACN, Task Force on Academic Progression, 2020a). "Quality patient care hinges on having a well-educated nursing workforce. Research has shown that lower mortality rates, fewer medication errors, and positive outcomes are all linked to nurses prepared at the baccalaureate and graduate degree levels" (AACN, n.d.).

Many organizations continue to oppose the law, including The Association of Community College Trustees (ACCT, 2017). The association believes their role is to address critical nursing shortages, specifically in rural locations, long-term care, and underserved populations. ACCT (2017) states there is no evidence that associate degree nurses are not fully prepared to fulfill their job responsibilities. ACCT (2017) also denies the broad statement that a baccalaureate education better prepares nurses for practice.

The AACN (2000) position statement supports higher education, affirming that a baccalaureate education should be the minimum entry-level preparation for professional nursing practice. The AACN has always fully supported ADN programs and has no intention to support the closure of such programs. They stand firm on not limiting the role of nurses educated at the ADN level, stating nurses should work in settings according to their type and level of education, reiterating the impact education has on skill and competency level. AACN (2019) believes ADN programs play a crucial role in meeting the healthcare needs of the nation. In addition, ". . . a sizeable majority of AACN members indicated support for RN licensure at the ADN level within the context of different scopes of practice for nurses based on level of education" (AACN, 2019, para. 3).

Incentives and Barriers for Earning a BSN

There are a number of reasons why nurses are returning to school to earn their BSN. One major incentive came from the IOM (2011) report, *The Future of Nursing. Leading Change, Advancing Health.* The report urged nurses in all settings to work collaboratively to increase the proportion of baccalaureate prepared nurses to 80% by 2020. Altmann (2011) reviewed 28 research studies that evaluated the incentives and barriers for nurses returning to school for a baccalaureate degree:

Incentives:

- Organizational incentives
- Personal achievement
- Desire for more nursing knowledge
- Job security
- Pressure from employer
- Ability to earn credit for past experience

Barriers:

- Multiple competing priorities in nurses' lives
- Working full-time
- Lack of confidence
- Feeling secure in a job
- Perceiving the baccalaureate degree as not enhancing clinical skills
- Perceiving baccalaureate prepared nurses as no different or not better (even inferior to) than those with less education
- Lack of credit for pre-licensure coursework or past experience
- Practical issues (inflexible or long programs)
- No increase in salary
- Different treatment at work
- Perceived lack of value
- Work schedules/conflicts/constraints; shift work
- Lack of support (financial or emotional) or recognition
- Having multiple roles or other responsibilities
- Length of time to complete the program; programs too long

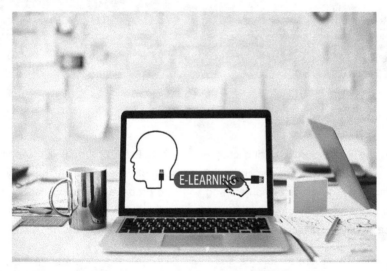

The IOM report (2011) has influenced the direction of nursing education and practice by disseminating the challenges and complexities of healthcare delivery in the 21st century. This leads into the next chapter, Healthcare in the 21st Century, which delves into the complexity of healthcare and how nursing practice continues to evolve.

Healthcare in the 21st Century

The need for a highly educated nursing workforce is in high demand due to the changing healthcare environment and the demographics of the U.S. population. Nurses require specialized knowledge and competencies to navigate the healthcare delivery system, such as leadership, research, integration of innovative technology and working in expanded roles and settings. These and other essential skill sets are vital for providing safe, high quality care. Nursing education and practice needs to move towards a patient-centered philosophy, higher standards for safe, quality care, with a stronger emphasis on information technology, scientific research, evidence-based practice, and interprofessional collaboration (Institute of Medicine [IOM], 2011).

The structure of America's healthcare environment has changed and will continue to evolve over time. Changing demographics brings about new cultures and practices. These cultural changes have brought about many questions about nursing's ability to adapt yet maintain core values. How can essential nursing values hold up in the rapidly changing 21st century? In order to better understand the need for adaptation, it is important to understand certain changes that occurred since the 1960s.

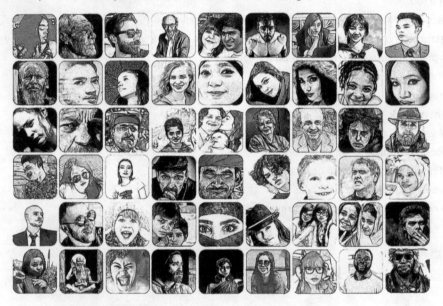

BSN Essentials

As previously discussed in the Professional Nursing chapter, the BSN Essentials outline the competencies of professional nursing practice. Essential IV, Information Management and Application of Patient Care Technology, states nurses must have a basic competence in technical skills (such as computers and software programs) and application of patient care technologies (such as monitors and data gathering technology). Additionally, nurses must be competent in information technology systems so they can gather evidence to guide practice (American Association of Colleges of Nursing [AACN], 2008).

Information literacy is crucial for the future of nursing, and healthcare system as a whole. McNeil, Elfrink, Beyea, Pierce, and Bickford (2006) explain the integration of evidence-based practice, interprofessional care coordination, and use of electronic health records rely on information management and technology to contain costs and improve safety (AACN, 2008).

Additional information about the Essentials can be found in the BSN Essentials document.

Immigration and Globalization

In the 20th and 21st century, immigrants from Europe, Africa, Central America and Asia continued to settle in the U.S. to escape war, poverty, and oppression. America gave them the chance to live free and practice their cultural and religious beliefs without fear of outright persecution. People have always come to America to seek out a better life for themselves and their children.

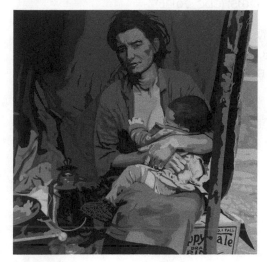

One effect of globalization is increased mobility and the advent of international aid programs to facilitate movement throughout the world (Bruce, 2018). Modern America's recent history was influenced by an immigration characterized by a mixture of religions, cultures, ethnicities, and races. Immigration from non-European areas has led to a wider variety of cultural integration becoming more pronounced in the U.S. (Bruce, 2018).

As a result of immigration and globalization, nurses must be committed to practice in a culturally congruent manner. According to the American Nurses Association (ANA, 2015c) Standards of Professional Performance, Standard 8, Culturally Congruent Practice, is fundamental to nursing practice.

Providing culturally congruent care begins with creating a personal inventory of one's values, beliefs, and cultural heritage (ANA, 2015c). Knowing oneself helps nurses understand themselves better, they may find more similarities than differences when reflecting on one's values and beliefs. Understanding the impact of discrimination and oppression on one's health helps nurses better understand their patients' needs, leading to a more accurate assessment and plan of care (ANA, 2015c).

Changing Demographics of the U.S.

As a result of immigration and globalization, the U.S. population has become more racially and culturally diverse. People are living longer with more chronic and complex illnesses as a result of technology and innovation. The following U.S. Census data (Colby & Ortman, 2015) projects an aging and more diverse U.S. population over the next 40 years:

- Increase from 319 million in 2014 to 417 million in 2060
- By 2030, one in five Americans is projected to be 65 and over
- By 2044, more than half of all Americans are projected to belong to a minority group (meaning any group other than non-Hispanic White)
- By 2060, nearly one in five of the nation's total population is projected to be foreign born

Nurses need to be aware of these changes, and be prepared to understand the differences with morality, and prevent bias. Language translation is just one aspect of accommodating our unique patient needs. As yourself, what other barriers will occur as a result of increasing cultural diversity?

Chronic Disease and Risk Factors

The leading cause of death in the U.S. is transitioning from infectious, acute disease to chronic and degenerative illnesses (Centers for Disease Control and Prevention [CDC], 2003). In addition to higher rates of chronic disease, the aging population leads to severe disability later in life.

- Chronic disease (2015): (at least two diagnoses): 67.7% of those ≥ 65 (CDC, 2018b)
- Obesity (2018): 30.9% (CDC, 2020c)

- Diabetes (2018)
    - Type I and II, diagnosed and undiagnosed: 34.1 million
        - Diagnosed: 26.8 million
        - Undiagnosed: 7.3 million (CDC, 2020b)
- Cardiovascular disease: 12.1% or 30.3 million (CDC, 2019)
- Arthritis, rheumatoid arthritis, gout, lupus, or fibromyalgia: 23% or 54 million (2015) (CDC, 2018b)

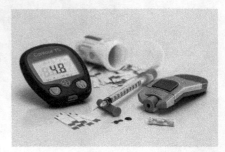

Chronic disease prevention and management requires individuals to modify risk factors that lead to chronic disease. The U.S. data below for adults aged 18 and older lists three modifiable risk factors for health promotion and disease prevention. Below are the current data for U.S. adults:

- Smoking:
    - 16.6% (2018)(CDC, 2018b)
    - 14% (2017)(CDC, 2018b)
    - 15.5% (2016) (CDC, 2018b)
    - 20.9% (2005) (CDC, 2020c)
- Exercise*(2017): 50% (CDC, 2020a)
- Diet (2017):
    - 36%: eats less than one fruit/day
    - 19%: eats less than one vegetable/day (CDC, 2020a)

* at least 150 minutes a week of moderate-intensity aerobic physical activity or 75 minutes a week of vigorous-intensity aerobic physical activity each week.

Technology and Healthcare

The 21st Century is known as the age of information technology. Healthcare has seen significant progress with technology and innovation over the past 25 years, especially since the Internet permeated almost every aspect of personal and work life. As a result, technology, specifically smartphones, has changed the way we interact with each other and how information is exchanged.

The following is a summary of the benefits of technological advances in healthcare:

- Improved effectiveness and efficiency
- Convenience (such as telehealth visit)
- Provide healthcare to rural locations, those with limited access to transportation (Huston, 2013)
- Data transparency
- Improved work environment, improved workflow
- Eliminates redundancy and duplication of documentation
- Reduces errors
- Eliminates interruptions for missing supplies, equipment, and medication
- Easier access to data
- Allows more time to spend with patients (as cited in Institute of Medicine, 2010)

Emerging Technologies

Huston (2013) cites the following emerging technologies that have a variety of benefits and challenges:

- **Genetics and Genomics**
  - Prenatal/newborn screening
  - Predictive value for disease or mutation
- **Less Invasive and More Accurate Tools for Diagnostics and Treatment**
  - Blood tests diagnose heart disease compared to diagnostic angiograms
  - Tattoos monitoring blood glucose without a finger stick
- **3-D Printing**
  - 3D printing of a prosthetic limbs, jaw, ear
- **Robotics**
  - Nanotechnology to prevent and treat disease
  - Pancreas pacemakers for diabetics
  - Miniature cameras and microphones that can be wired into the brain, will exist, allowing blind people to see and deaf people to hear
- **Biometrics**
  - Biometric signatures (fingerprints, retinal scan, voice recognition, etc.) improve confidentiality and security of data
- **Electronic Healthcare Records (EHR)**
  - Captures data to improve safety and quality of care
- **Computerized Physician/Provider Order; Entry (CPOE) and Clinical Decision Support**
  - Electronic orders lead to enhance healthcare decision-making and actions (pp. 3-10)

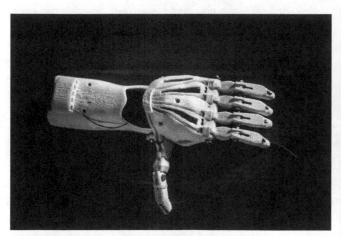 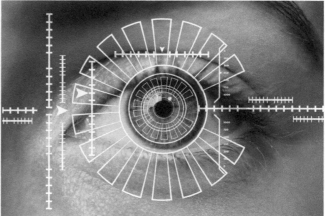

The Human Connection

Huston (2013) explains the core challenges with technology, such as retaining the human element in practice (discussed below). Balancing the high cost of technology with the benefits is significant for the entire healthcare system, including hospitals, clinics, pharmacies, etc. Initial training of the nursing workforce with ongoing competency is costly, compelling leadership to find ways to contain these high costs. Lastly, ensuring technology is used in an ethical way has become increasingly important with the advent of lifesaving technology and even integration of robots. Do patient want to check into their provider's office by speaking to a robot? Technology can bring about fear of the unknown when a new treatment is touted to cure disease beyond what is normally possible.

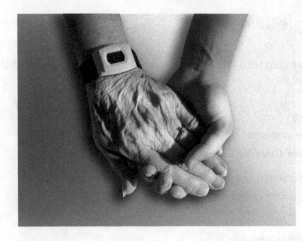

Technology can improve the quality of one's life in many circumstances, though it can also bring on ethical questions. Is it worth prolonging one's life to the point where quality is reduced or no longer exists?

Healthcare as we know it today is heavily reliant on technology to streamline care, though innovation has isolated nurses and other healthcare staff from interacting with patients in a number of ways. Consider self-registration and automatic check-in stations. As much as technology can save time and be more cost-effective, the loss of the personal touch can negatively impact healthcare. The loss of a human connection, social cues, and rich conversations negatively impact care by inadvertently fragmenting care and a disconnecting the patient from the healthcare team (Thorne et al., 2005).

Innovation increases the risk of losing sight of the core values that are the inherent in the nursing profession (Lee, Laux, & Robitaille, 2018). Nurses are challenged to fit in the time to nurture the human connection with patients, coworkers and other support staff. Nurses need to find creative, personal ways outside of technology to show caring and compassion, especially in stressful work environments like healthcare settings.

How often do patients receive full eye contact during an intake? Technology can save time and resources, though it can cause patients to feel like a number (Thorne et al., 2005).

Medical breakthroughs, technological advances, and experimental treatments can also give patients a false sense of security that disease can be cured (Lee et al., 2018). For example, patients may struggle to know when it is the right time to end cancer treatments. Innovative treatments can offer endless treatment options, requiring nurses to assist patients with these important decisions. Providing the caring and compassion outside the veil of technology should encourage nurses to be fully present.

The Changing Role of Nursing Practice

The foundational report by the IOM (2010), *The Future of Nursing: Leading Change, Advancing Health,* asserts that nurses are poised to play a critical role in transforming the healthcare system to meet the increasing demands for safe, high-quality, accessible, and cost-effective healthcare. In order to provide this high level of care, nurses at all levels of care must understand how they can be involved in this momentous change. Such changes require nurses to consider a new way of thinking and practicing. Instead of providing care with the focus on the disease process, nurses need to view the bigger picture, and transition towards promoting care across the continuum. The patient's family must be considered within the community setting to ensure the needed supports and resources are accessible, leading to health and well-being (Salmond & Echevarria, 2017).

Salmond and Echevarria (2017) review four core areas of nursing practice necessary for improving care:

- Wellness
- Patient- and family-centered care
- Care coordination
- Data analytics; focus on outcomes and improvement

Nurses need to transition care from an illness-based focus to one that incorporates prevention and wellness approaches (Salmond & Echevarria, 2017). Prevention strategies must begin at home and within the community in order to maintain health and well-being. Nurses are uniquely positioned to educate patients and their families about the role of health promotion and self-care in preventing acute illnesses.

Social Determinants of Health

Thinking beyond the acute care event is an integral part of a complete patient assessment. Considering the factors leading up to an acute illness are often a combination of both social and environmental triggers. These triggers, such as living in a safe neighborhood and health literacy, will influence nurses' decision-making throughout the entire nursing process. See Table 1 for a list of environmental and social triggers, known as social and physical determinants of health (U.S. Department of Health and Human Services, 2020). Nurses must be cognizant of the changing demographics of the U.S. population when considering the determinants of health throughout all aspects of care.

Table 1 depicts the social and physical determinants of health

Table 1: Social and Physical Determinants of Health *by Healthy People 2020*

Social Determinants	Environmental (physical) Determinants
Availability of resources to meet daily needs (e.g., safe housing and local food markets)	Natural environment, such as green space (e.g., trees and grass) or weather (e.g., climate change)
Access to educational, economic, and job opportunities	Built environment, such as buildings, sidewalks, bike lanes, and roads
Access to health care services	Worksites, schools, and recreational settings
Quality of education and job training	Housing and community design
Availability of community-based resources in support of community living and opportunities for recreational and leisure-time activities	Exposure to toxic substances and other physical hazards
Transportation options	Physical barriers, especially for people with disabilities
Public safety	Aesthetic elements (e.g., good lighting, trees, and benches)
Social support	
Social norms and attitudes (e.g., discrimination, racism, and distrust of government)	
Exposure to crime, violence, and social disorder (e.g., presence of trash and lack of cooperation in a community)	
Socioeconomic conditions (e.g., concentrated poverty and the stressful conditions that accompany it)	
Residential segregation	
Language/Literacy	
Access to mass media and emerging technologies (e.g., cell phones, the Internet, and social media)	
Culture	
	(U.S. Department of Health and Human Services, 2018)

Alvarado (2019) studied the relationship between childhood neighborhoods and whether there was a relationship to adult obesity. The results found children were more likely to be obese during adulthood when exposed to disadvantaged neighborhoods. While nurses need to instill the public health message of curbing obesity in adulthood, awareness of factors that lead to obesity must be considered. According to this study, policy needs to focus on the processes that occur during childhood development, such as the state of the neighborhoods where children live and play.

Patient- and family-centered care intersects with care coordination as a result of nursing's strong emphasis on providing holistic care. Delivering holistic care ensures an unwavering focus on the needs of the patient and family (American Nurses Association, 2012). Advocating for and embracing patients and families as active partners in their care is integral for providing quality care. Nurses need to acknowledge that patients' input is invaluable and must include patients and families as partners in decision-making. When patients and families are part of the decision-making process, they become more vested in their care, they are incentivized to meet self-care needs and follow through with disease prevention activities (Salmond & Echevarria, 2017).

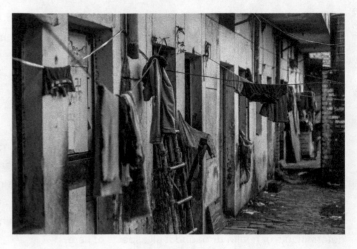

An essential part of reaching health outcomes and improved quality of care relies on nurses understanding the care they provide. Nurses need to recognize that data influences their care, and healthcare delivery as a whole. Understanding key metrics, such as hospital readmissions or infection rates, is an example of how data informs practice. Nurses need to use data to improve practice at the individual level, though understanding the data at the population level is how practice evolves (Salmond & Echevarria, 2017). Through collaboration with other disciplines and researchers, nurses are able to use data to reach new goals to improve outcomes and quality, reduce cost, and more.

Upholding Nurses Values

As the configuration of America's communities change as a result of globalization, nurses must stay true to their core values of caring for others for altruistic reasons. Many nurses enter the profession due to their desire to help and care for others in need. Nurses are faced with providing care to a changing demographic, having to understand and respect the most vulnerable patients with human dignity (Bruce, 2018).

Nurses are caring for patients who fled their countries due to violence, sexual assault, and religious persecution, hoping to live in America's communities. Patients are relying on nurses to protect them, care for them without bias or prejudice, both emotionally and physically. Nurses have the power to ensure quality care to these vulnerable patients. Nurses are no stranger to advocating for patients' needs, though practice must continually adapt in this changing environment.

Bruce (2018) writes about the importance of nurses upholding and actively maintaining the core values of why nurses entered this beloved and amazing profession. Providing care in a selfless, noble way is still a primary mission of nurses, and when these values are combined with a caring approach, nurses are well prepared to support diversity and meet patients' healthcare needs. Increasing tolerance will lead nurses to embrace the differences that are encountered when patients have opposing beliefs, different ethnicities, races, religion, sexual orientation, and citizenship. Caring for vulnerable populations requires the core value of caring for every kind of patient to be a prominent aspect of all nursing practice.

In order to ensure healthcare delivery offers safe, high quality, and cost-effective care, nurses must assume diverse roles and achieve a wide variety of competencies (knowledge, skills, abilities). Nurses play a central role in transforming care at the individual level, and when nurses work together, change can occur broadly, for broader community. Below is a brief review of the necessary roles and competencies of the nursing workforce for the 21st Century:

- Change agent
- Lead and inspire others towards change
- Disease prevention and wellness
- Prevention of adverse events (such as hospital-acquired infections)
- Clinical knowledge grounded in evidence

- Respond to data and track trends
- Focus on excellence and the patient experience
- Responsiveness to determinants of health
- Management of chronic conditions
- Care coordination across the continuum
- Patient-centric, patient as a partner
- Team-based, collaborative care
- Optimize the use of innovative technology
- Patient and family advocacy to promote:
- health promotion
- navigation of a complex healthcare systems

Accountability

Accountability is foundational to professional nursing practice and is often referred to as the "hallmark of professionalism" (Oyetunde & Brown, 2012). Being accountable can be described in a few ways. According to the American Nurses Association (ANA, 2015), nursing accountability requires nurses to be answerable for their actions and act according to a code of ethical conduct. Such ethical conduct includes abiding by the principles of beneficence, respect for human dignity, veracity, fidelity, loyalty, and patient autonomy. See the content below on the *Code of Ethics* for the impact accountability has on nursing practice.

Leonenko and Drach-Zahavy (2016) describe how professional accountability impacts all aspects of patient care, such as activities of daily living, health promotion, patient teaching, counseling, and collaboration with the interprofessional team (provider, therapy, dietician, etc.). While some education may not be provided by the nurse, such as mobility exercises from physical therapy, it is the nurse's responsibility to ensure all services and education are in place and monitored throughout care. Accountable nurses will focus on instilling the patients trust in not only oneself, but the nursing profession as a whole. Patients can earn the trust of the profession when they see team cohesiveness, collaboration, and nurses working together towards a common goal (Leonenko & Drach-Zahavy, 2016).

Accountability can be seen throughout all aspects of nursing practice, such as:

- Ensuring/providing safe, quality care
- Delegation
- Following (and questioning) policy and procedures
- Practicing within the guidelines of the Nurse Practice Act
- Maintaining confidentiality
- Questioning standard of care, provider's orders
- Alignment of care to organizational practices, philosophy
- Competence in clinical skills
- Lifelong learning
- Patient advocacy (Battié, & Steelman, 2014)

Accountability is a broad concept that is closely related to other concepts. It will be important to understand the differences between the following concepts as they are discussed throughout this chapter:

- **Accountability**:
    - Judgment and action on the part of the nurse
    - Answerable to self and others for judgments and actions (ANA, 2015a)
- **Responsibility**:
    - Accountability or liability associated with performance of a nursing task associated with one's role
    - Portion of the responsibility can be shared with others involved in the situation (ANA, 2015a)
- **Answerability**:
    - The requirement to offer answers, rationale, and explanations (ANA, 2015a)
- **Authority**:
    - The position to make a decision and influence others to act
- **Autonomy**:
    - the authority to use professional knowledge and judgment to make decisions and take action (Skår, 2009)

Cox and Beeson (2018) describe accountability as a "... a willingness to answer for results and behavior" (p. 25). When nurses are accountable for their actions, they have made a promise to own that action, leading to learning lessons from making mistakes and successes. People don't hold others accountable, it's the individual's job to be accountable.

In today's healthcare settings, accountability in nursing practice revolves around activities associated with providing quality care, including:

- Assessments (patients or otherwise, depending on setting/role)
- Interventions (nursing care)
- Health outcomes (reduced infection rates, falls)
- Costs (containment)

Many organizations, both federal and private, have created programs to improve the quality of healthcare, including the U.S. Agency for Healthcare Research and Quality, The Joint Commission, National Patient Safety Goals, and the Institute for Healthcare Improvement. The Institute of Medicine (IOM) and Quality and Safety Education for Nurses Institute (QSEN) are two organizations focused on safety in nursing education. Scientific evidence reveals the gap in quality care and these organizations (and others) work from different vantage points inside and outside of the healthcare system to reduce the incidence of unsafe, poor quality care.

Transfer of accountability from one nurse to another is like a silent contract. For example, in an acute care setting, when a nurse receives report from the outgoing nurse, there is a transfer of accountability from one person to another. The oncoming nurse is responsible and answerable for the behaviors and outcomes of a group of patients for the duration of the shift. Thus, anytime a nurse establishes a professional relationship with a patient (depending on role/setting), there is a binding agreement where the nurse is legally bound (see Nurse Practice Act below) to implement care according to the patient's needs and wishes.

State Boards of Nursing

As mentioned earlier, accountability within the nursing profession ensures safe, quality care. In order to protect the public and to ensure optimum care, nursing practice is regulated by state agencies. The U.S. Boards of Nursing (BON) are jurisdictional governmental agencies that have been established by each state government with the mission to protect the public's health by overseeing nursing practice (National Council of State Boards of Nursing [NCSBN], 2020a).

The NCSBN (2020a) administers and coordinates services to all state BONs. The NCSBN works with each state BON to ensure nursing accountability through a number of organizational activities, including standards for safe nursing practice, issuing licenses to practice nursing, license verification, monitoring licensees' compliance to state BON laws, and taking action against nurses who have exhibited unsafe nursing practice (NCSBN, 2020a).

Nurse Practice Act

Individual states, or jurisdictions, have a law called the nurse practice act (NPA), which is enforced by the BON in each state (NCSBN, 2020a). The NPA includes the following information:

- Qualifications for licensure
- Nursing titles that can be used
- Scope of practice (what the nurse is allowed to do)
- Actions that can or will occur if nurses do not follow the laws

The scope of practice is in place to safeguard patient care and maximize health outcomes. When nurses practice outside of their scope of practice, accountability to oneself, the patient/family, peers, the institution, and/or society are at risk. Familiarity with the NPA ensures accountability.

Access the NPA for New York at the Office of the Professions (OOP) website, located within the New York State Education Department. A number of articles and information about the nursing profession are available at the OOP, including laws about scope of practice, nursing education, education curricula/programs, disciplinary conduct, and more. Read Part 64 at the Office of the Professions (OOP) website to view the scope of practice for the registered nurse.

Nurses should review their NPA regularly to check for updates, and most importantly, when changing jobs or taking on a formal leadership role. Laws within the NPA pertain to certain settings and roles. For a full listing of all the NPAs in every state, visit the NCSBN website.

Foundational Documents

Standards of Professional Practice

Accountability is an essential element of nursing practice within the Scope and Standards of Practice. Below are a few examples where accountability and responsibility for nursing practice are illustrated throughout the Standards of Professional Performance.

- **Standard 7: Ethics**
  - "Demonstrates professional **accountability and responsibility** for nursing" practice (ANA, 2015c, p. 67).
- **Standard 10: Collaboration**
  - "Clearly articulates the nurse's role and **responsibilities** within the team" (ANA, 2015c, p. 73).
- **Standard 11: Leadership**
  - "Retains accountability for delegated nursing care" (ANA, 2015c, p. 75).
- **Standard 15: Professional Practice Evaluation**
  - "Ensures that nursing practice is consistent with regulatory requirements pertaining to licensure, relevant statutes, rules, and regulations" (ANA, 2015c, p. 81).
  - "Uses organizational policies and procedures to guide professional practice" (ANA, 2015c, p. 81).
  - "Delegates in accordance with applicable legal and policy parameters" (ANA, 2015c, p. 81).

Nursing's Social Policy Statement

Nursing's social policy statement describes nursing's social responsibility, accountability and contribution to healthcare (ANA, 2015b). The nursing profession is entrusted with providing quality, ethical care to society. The ANA is responsible for ensuring societies' needs are met by articulating, maintaining, and strengthening the social contracts between the nursing profession and society.

Code of Ethics

The (ANA, 2015a) *Code of Ethics* sets forth the values and obligations of the nurse. Provision 4 has a core focus on accountability and responsibility, stating, "The nurse has authority, accountability, and responsibility for nursing practice; makes decisions; and takes action consistent with the obligation to promote health and to provide optimal care" (ANA, 2015a, p. 59). The nurse's ethical obligation is to protect and be accountable to oneself, and also to the general public.

The following four interpretive statements from Provision 4 further illustrate the depth of accountability and responsibility in nursing practice:

4.1 Authority, Accountability, and Responsibility

- Accountable for one's own practice, care ordered by a provider, care coordination.

4.2 Accountability for Nursing Judgments, Decisions, and Actions

- Nurses must follow a code of ethical conduct.
- Follow the scope and standards of nursing practice.

4.3 Responsibility for Nursing Judgments, Decisions, and Action

- The nurse is always accountable for judgments, decisions, and actions, though the employer may be jointly responsible depending on the situation.
- Nurses accept or reject an assignment based on education, experience, competence, and risk for patient safety.

4.4 Assignment and Delegation of Nursing Activities or Tasks

- Assignments and delegation activities must be consistent with the Nurse Practice Act, organizational policy, and nursing standards of practice.
- Assess individual competence prior to assigning (ANA, 2015a, p. 59).

BSN Essentials

The BSN Essentials illustrate the outcomes for baccalaureate nursing education (AACN, 2008). Accountability and responsibility are a major component of the nine essentials, see below for more information:

- **Assumptions of a Baccalaureate Generalist Nurse**
    - Assume **accountability** for one's own and delegated nursing care
- **Roles for the Baccalaureate Generalist Nurse**
    - The use of the term "professional" implies the formation of a professional identity and **accountability** for one's professional image
- **Essential II: Basic Organizational and Systems Leadership for Quality Care and Patient Safety**
    - Apply leadership concepts, skills, and decision making in the provision of high quality nursing care, healthcare team coordination, and the oversight and **accountability** for care delivery in a variety of settings
- **Essential VI: Interprofessional Communication and Collaboration for Improving Patient Health Outcomes**
    - Individual accountability/shared accountability
- **Essential VIII: Professionalism and Professional Values**
    - Professionalism involves **accountability** for oneself and nursing practice, including continuous professional engagement and lifelong learning
- **Essential IX: Baccalaureate Generalist Nursing Practice**
    - Demonstrate clinical judgment and **accountability** for patient outcomes when delegating to and supervising other members of the healthcare team (AACN, 2008).

More information can be found in the BSN Essentials document.

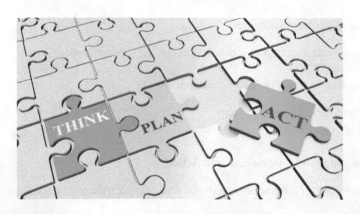

Types of Accountability

Nurses are accountable for their actions to themselves, their peers, employer, healthcare consumers, society, and the nursing profession (ANA, 2015c).

Accountability to Self

Nurses must be accountable to themselves, otherwise they risk accountability to their peers and their patients. Nurses work very long hours, often working well past a 12-hour shift to complete care, documentation, and report to the oncoming nurse. A nurse may resent having to work a 13- or 14-hour shift, especially when compensation may not cover the extra time on the unit. Miller (2012) explains the importance of strengthening personal accountability in situations where a nurse may begin complaining or blaming others about the long hours or other issues that are beyond the nurse's control. Personal accountability begins with looking inward, rather than pointing fingers. Miller (2012) suggests asking oneself two important questions:

- What can I do?
- How can I help?

Instead of just complaining to the manager about the long shift or a different problem, nurses need to offer their assistance on how to find a resolution and offer their help with carrying out the solution. Part of resolving problems is being part of the solution. Nurses who refuse to complain, and instead choose to find solutions, become empowered. Choosing to be positive, and part of the solution, leads to improving one's personal accountability.

As previously mentioned, working long hours in a stressful environment requires nurses to have adequate physical stamina and emotional stability. Fatigue, minor illnesses, and a stressful personal life can negatively impact professional practice. Working extra shifts in addition to a very busy life can also hamper practice. Maintaining a healthy lifestyle, including adequate sleep, diet, and exercise, and having a balanced work-personal life, is essential for one's personal accountability.

Working in an unsafe practice setting is another example where nurses need to be accountable to themselves. Some examples include working in an unfamiliar setting or having a high-acuity/high patient load assignment. Nurses need to view refusal to work in an unsafe setting as a way to protect the public, and to be personally accountable. Be sure to follow organizational policies on how to refuse and/or make a statement about working in an unsafe environment.

Accountability to Peers

Accountability to peers is also known as shared accountability. Shared accountability occurs when team members support each other, work together to ensure a safe working environment, and act as role models to demonstrate a culture of respect. If nurses need to speak up about a concern, they need to do so in a constructive, considerate way. Communication with team members should be provided consistently, in a way that does not cause embarrassment or anger. When team members consistently share feedback with each other it reinforces the desire for a supportive, cohesive team. The goal is to create an environment where suggestions for change are expected and become the norm. Establishing a culture of trust, respect, and support leads to a healthy work environment and quality safe patient care (Battié, & Steelman, 2014).

Accountability to the Employer

Nurses are accountable to their employers by following their rules and regulations and fulfilling their job duties. Since nurses must be accountable with the laws set forth in the NPA, they need to verify organization policies do not conflict with NPA regulations. Nurses risk violating regulations if they do not review the NPA regularly. Nurses are also responsible, and held accountable, for monitoring unlicensed personnel. Nurses can improve accountability to their employer by taking an active role in organization-wide committees focused on improving the delivery of care.

Accountability to the Patient

Patients have the right to safe, quality care. Nurses are held accountable to their patient by the fulfilling their obligations set for in the *Scope and Standards of Practice* and the *Code of Ethics*. As previously stated, these two foundational documents illustrate the requirement of all registered nurses to provide exemplary care to individuals in need of healthcare.

Nurses can also be accountable to their patients by educating them about the Hospital Compare website. All hospitals are now required to post health outcomes and other measures at the Hospital Compare website so patients can make choices about where to receive care. Visit the Hospital Compare website to view all of the outcomes. The following is a brief list of the outcomes found in the Hospital Compare website:

- Timely and effective care
- Healthcare associated infections (HAI)
- Adverse effects (i.e. mortality rates)
- Patient satisfaction/experiences

The quality measures available from the Hospital Compare website provides the healthcare system and nurses important data that helps them be more competitive with other healthcare systems, thus, further improving quality care. Nurses need to be aware their patients often enter the healthcare system with increased knowledge of healthcare in general and awareness of the organization's level of quality care. Patients may have a sense of what to expect from nurses when they begin receiving care, and nurses must be prepared to work with patients in a collaborative way. Like any other business, healthcare organizations and their employees must be accountable to their patients and their needs.

Since the healthcare system has moved towards a proactive, preventive care approach, nurses need to provide patients with the education and tools to promote health and well-being in order to prevent illness and disease. As nurses develop relationships with their patients, it will be important to understand their distinct needs and how they relate to health promotion activities. For example, determining any barriers and motivating factors will be important for nurses to include in their collaborative efforts with patients. When nurses create a plan that is patient-centered, and focused on current evidence to offer safe, quality care, nurses are taking the right steps to being accountable to their patients.

Accountability to Society

One of the characteristics of a profession is service to society. Consumers have the right to receive safe, quality care, and nurses are held accountable to meet the healthcare needs of society. To meet these needs and requirements, nurses are obligated to stay abreast of current literature, attain continuing education, maintain skill competencies, and more. Through the NPA and the ANA's *Nursing's Social Policy Statement*, nurses are legally held accountable to provide professional nursing care that meets the required scopes and standards of practice.

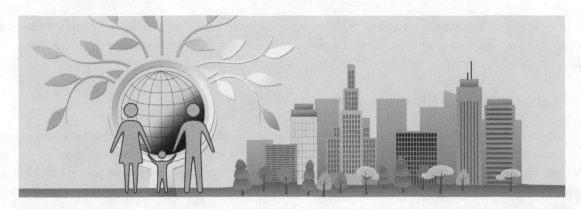

Accountability to the Nursing Profession

Just as nurses are advocates for their patients, they must also be strong advocates for the nursing profession. Through participation in professional nursing organizations, nurses need to promote safe, quality nursing care, improved nursing autonomy, nurses' rights, and more. Nurses need to support professional organizations as a way to be accountable to the nursing profession (Battié, & Steelman, 2014). Nurses can demonstrate their accountability by the following activities:

- Participate in organization-sponsored conferences and activities
- Stay current with recommended practices within one's specialty
- Political advocacy
- Vote for candidates who support the profession's mission (Battié, & Steelman, 2014)

Nurses play an important role in shaping the nursing profession through formulating its own policies and laws. Nurses work collaboratively to formulate the profession's scope, standards of care, licensing, entry into practice, and more.

Provision 3 in the ANA (2015a) *Code of Ethics* states, "The nurse promotes, advocates for, and protects the rights, health, and safety of the patient" (p. 41). Interpretive statement 3.5 explains how nurses must act on questionable practice. Nurses must be alert to all instances of incompetent, unethical, illegal, or impaired practice by another member of the healthcare team, which includes issues that occur within the entire healthcare system. Nurses must take action to resolve such issues in order to protect the healthcare consumer from injustice or injury.

The *Code of Ethics* directs nurses not only to recognize questionable practice due to impairment, such as substance abuse, but nurses are also obligated with assisting each other with obtaining treatment. Weber (2017) states substance and alcohol abuse is a significant issue for the nursing profession. Chemically addicted nurses and other healthcare workers pose a danger to themselves, patients, team members, and the organization.

Manthey (2018) discusses how nurses are at an increased risk for addiction due to working in highly stressful environments, easy access to highly addictive substances, and a "conspiracy of silence" that prevents treatment. Thomas and Siela (2011) states at least 1 in 10 nurses will develop a substance abuse disorder, similar to the general public. Resources and more information about substance abuse disorders in nurses can be found at the NCSBN website.

Nurses must be acutely aware of the high risk of addiction to alcohol and illegal substances for oneself. When nurses observe impaired practice or unsafe patient care from a coworker and believe wrongdoing has occurred (such as drug-diverting), nurses must be prepared to report this unethical behavior. Reporting such behaviors to authorities is known as whistleblowing. Whistleblowing is defined as "the disclosure by organisation members (former or current) of illegal, immoral or illegitimate practices under the control of their employers, to persons or organizations that may be able to effect action" (Near & Miceli, 1985, p. 4). Protecting patients from harm is one of the guiding principles of the nursing profession. Nurses owe it to themselves, and their patients to ensure be alert to impaired practice and reporting such behaviors. Additional information about whistleblowing can be found at the ANA website.

Nurses can advocate for their profession by supporting their peers who struggle with alcohol or substance abuse. Nurses can recommend their peers seek assistance from a program run by the New York State Nurses Association called the Statewide Peer Assistance for Nurses (SPAN, 2018) program. SPAN services are available to all nurses working in New York State. SPAN offers nurses assistance with substance abuse including other confidential services, such as education, support, and advocacy. Additional information on helping nurses with addiction can be found at the SPAN website.

In order to ensure the nursing profession continues to be known as an honorable and noble profession, nurses need to support and mentor their peers throughout one's career.

Nursing Judgment and Action

Nurses practice and act within a learned code of ethics they implicitly follow when making judgments about care. Nurses practice by the principle of fidelity (being faithful, honest), respect for dignity, work, and patient autonomy when taking action. Nurses are accountable for judgments made about care. When nurses assume accountability and responsibility for their patients, they fulfill their commitment to practice with compassion and respect for patients. The ANA (2010a) states, "The moral standard of the profession is one to which nurses must hold themselves and their peers in order to be held accountable in for their practice" (p. 46).

Nurses must either reject or accept role demands based on one's level of education, knowledge, competence, and experience. Nurses must assess their own competencies and seek out necessary education, consultation, and collaboration. Tasks should be performed only when nurses have demonstrated sufficient competence and confidence with the skill.

When nurses are answerable for their knowledge, skills, and actions, their level of respect and nursing autonomy grows. The general public needs nurses to be competent; therefore, when nurses demonstrate their strengths by providing competent care, they maintain the trust and respect of their patients including the healthcare system as a whole.

As described earlier, autonomy is centered around nurses making independent decisions about care based on their knowledge, judgment, and experience. Autonomy is related to accountability because nurses who make independent decisions, or any decision for that matter, are accountable for their actions. Autonomous decisions are made to ensure appropriate care, maintain high quality care, and satisfy the patient or healthcare consumer.

Shared Governance

Shared governance is an organizational model defined as "... a structure within the process of practicing professional nursing that results in favorable nurse, patient, and organizational outcomes" (Church, Baker, & Berry, 2008, p. 36). The two main assumptions of shared governance models are: 1) redistribute decision-making power from managers to staff [nurses], and 2) nurses have the interest in being part of the decision-making process (Anthony, 2004).

Golanowski, Beaudry, Kurz, Laffey, and Hook (2007) explains shared governance as a decision-making model containing four major concepts:

- **Accountability:** the foundational concept, includes authority (power to make decisions), autonomy (right to make independent decisions), and control (ability to act)
- **Equity:** measure of all team members contributions to the outcome
- **Partnership:** relationships among the team members with a focus on the outcome
- **Ownership:** invested in the organization, able to articulate personal contribution to the outcome

Shared governance can transform nurses' personal practice and benefit healthcare organizations in many ways, including:

- Empowerment of practice (Hess, 2004)
- Improved nurse satisfaction (Church et al., 2008; Golanowski et al., 2007)
- Improved patient satisfaction scores (Church et al., 2008)
- Reduced mortality and healthcare-acquired infection rates (Church et al., 2008)
- Reduced nurse turnover and vacancy rates (Church et al., 2008)
- Improved staff morale (Golanowski et al., 2007)
- Improved staff member participation (Golanowski et al., 2007)
- Personal and professional development (Golanowski et al., 2007)

Improved levels of morale, job satisfaction, and empowerment leads nurses to being happier, and more fulfilled in their daily work. Patients can sense when their caregivers (nurses and staff members) exhibit more cheerful and contented behaviors, which may translate to feelings of being cared for, and having a satisfied patient experience.

In order for a shared governance model to bring about positive outcomes, both nurses and managers need to buy into the idea that nurses need to have a voice in decisions that impact their practice, and the delivery of healthcare.

Delegation

Delegation is defined as, "The transfer of responsibility for the performance of a task from one individual to another while retaining accountability for the outcome" (ANA, 2015c, p. 86). The ANA and NCSBN (2019) created the *Joint Statement on Delegation* in order to support and guide nurses on how to use delegation safely and effectively. These organizations share the following definition and meanings about delegation:

- The process for a nurse to direct another person to perform nursing tasks and activities. The nurse retains the accountability for the delegated task (ANA & NCSBN, 2019, para 3). The two organizations further delineate:
  - NCSBN: nurse transfers authority
  - ANA: nurse transfer of responsibility

Nurses often work in chaotic healthcare environments, have a large patient load, a high acuity assignment with complex patient needs, with an added emphasis on patient satisfaction. These are just a few factors that leave nurses no choice but to delegate tasks to other members of the healthcare team. Delegation frees up nurses' valuable time so nurses can attend to more complex patient care tasks. Delegation is an essential skill of professional nursing practice, and when done correctly, can result in safe and effective nursing care (ANA, 2019).

Delegation is an expectation and responsibility of nursing practice as identified in the ANA Standards of Professional Performance, Standard 15, Resource Utilization: "Delegates elements of care to appropriate healthcare workers in accordance with any applicable legal or policy parameters or principles" (ANA, 2015c, p. 81).

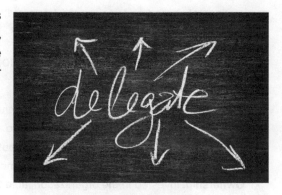

In order to delegate, nurses must consider the following:

- Nurses' legal authority to practice
- Context of their practice
- Nurse Practice Act regulations
- Professional standards
- Employer's policies and procedures on delegation (ANA, 2019)

More information about the ANA's *Principles for Delegation* and NCSBN's *Decision Tree for Delegation to Nursing Assistive Personnel* can be found in their the Joint Statement on Delegation document.

Creating a Culture of Accountability

It is essential to view accountability as a process of supporting others who want to be accountable for the work they accomplish. Nurses in leadership positions, whether formal (i.e. nurse manager) or informal (i.e. charge or staff nurse), should reflect on their thoughts about accountability in order to get a full understanding of one's thoughts on the topic. Reflection is an important first step because leaders set the tone for the work setting and understanding oneself better can impact thinking and actions for the future (Cox & Beeson, 2018). Some questions to consider include:

- Do you set a tone of learning from mistakes or do you focus on punishing?
- Do you focus on blaming others or fix the system?
- Are you the first or last to admit your own mistakes? (Cox & Beeson, 2018)

Providing support to individuals who make mistakes, rather than finding faults, will create an environment where accountability can grow. Enforcing a punitive consequence destroys the possibility of creating trust and a sense of partnership with a peer or follower. Accountability should be associated with support, encouragement, trust, and unquestionably, not punishment (Cox & Beeson, 2018).

Cox and Beeson (2018) explains the three major components of accountability:

- **Clear expectations**: clearly explain the expectations by answering the 4-Ws and the 1-H, such as:
  - **What** needs to be done?
  - **Why** is this important?
  - **When** does it need to be completed?
  - **Who** else will I be working with on the project?
  - **How** do I begin?
- **Follow-through**: connect with staff to offer motivation or inspiration to carry out the task or project:
  - Mentoring
  - Coaching
  - Guiding
  - Feedback
  - Encouragement
  - Support
- **Rewards or consequences**
  - Reward: A pat on the back when the task is complete. Be sincere and timely
  - Consequence: be firm and compassionate

Summary of How to Enhance Accountability

- Clear and open communication
- Skill competency
- Advanced education
- Collaboration with peers, managers
- Clear expectations
- Participate in professional organization opportunities
- Support peers, mentor new nurses, offer guidance

- Read the NPA regularly, especially when changing roles/settings
- Delegate
- Ask yourself, "What can I do? and "How can I help?"
- Maintain a healthy lifestyle; physically, emotionally, spiritually
- Choose to be positive, find a solution
- Participate in organization-wide committees
- Be compassionate, listen
- Organize a shared governance model for your unit/organization
- Compare employer's policies/processes to NPA

Autonomy

Autonomy is fundamental to nursing practice and it is one of the most essential characteristics of the profession. Autonomy is defined as the authority to use professional knowledge and judgment to make decisions and take action (Skår, 2009; Traynor, Boland, & Buus, 2010). Skår (2010) further defines nursing autonomy as "Authority of total patient care, the power to make decisions in a relationship with the patient and next of kin and the freedom to make clinical judgments, choices and actions ..." (p. 2233). Autonomy is also referred to as self-determination, self-direction, independence, and self-governance.

Skår (2009) found the following four themes from her research on finding the meaning of autonomy in nursing practice:

- to have a holistic view
- to know that you know
- to know the patient
- to dare (an expression of personal ability)

Types of Autonomy

Weston (2008) defines two types of autonomy in nursing practice:

1. **Clinical autonomy**: The authority, freedom, and discretion of nurses to make judgments about patient care
2. **Control over practice**: The authority, freedom, and discretion of nurses to make decisions related to the practice setting, such as the organizational structure, governance, rules, policies, and operations

Skår (2009) studied the meaning of nurses' experiences of autonomy in practice and found knowledge and confidence were the two major requirements for independent decision-making. Nurses begin exercising their clinical autonomy as their knowledge improves through experience and collaboration within the interdisciplinary team. As clinical competence improves, nurses gain the necessary confidence needed to make decisions about care.

Regardless of advanced knowledge and experience, nurses are bound to find themselves in a position where they are unprepared to complete a task. Skår (2009) found nurses will rely on their personal capabilities and confidence to figure out what they need to know and how to proceed. In addition, Skår (2009) found it takes personal courage to act, stating, "The nurses' confidence in *knowing that they know* as well as *knowing that they dare* is important for making autonomous clinical judgements and decisions" (p. 2232). In other words, nurses pull from their depth of knowledge and experience and use their courage to complete the task.

An example of clinical autonomy for a nurse who has begun to develop some competencies and advanced knowledge may start to question physician orders or share ideas about treatment options with the provider. The nurse may reflect on a conversation with a peer or recall a patient from the past that offers guidance and relevant information about care options. As Skår (2010) points out, patient care decisions are based on knowledge and confidence, therefore, as nurses develop their competencies and gain additional knowledge, independent decision-making will grow. The longer a nurse practices and acquires more competencies (i.e. wound care certificate), and new knowledge (i.e. specialty certification, advanced degrees), practice will continue to become more autonomous over time.

Nurses make autonomous decisions all the time, sometimes without realizing it. Consider the following practice examples nurses make on a regular basis in regard to clinical autonomy:

- Administer prn pain medication
- Raise the head of bed when a patient is short of breath
- Seek out the physical therapist to discuss advancing ambulation
- Request a dietician referral when assessments find poor wound healing
- Delegate aide to assist with ambulation
- Check blood sugar due to confusion and weakness

In order for nurses to exert control over their practice, they need to question whether the environment allows for autonomous practice. Below are some examples of how nurses can demonstrate control over their practice:

- Does the current policy on assessing tube feeding placement rely on current evidence-based practice?
- The supply room is always short of supplies. The nurse will inquire about the procedure for stocking the room and suggest ideas for improvement.
- Unit policies and procedures change without input from nursing staff. The nurse will speak with the manager about organizing a shared-governance approach for the unit, and possibly institution-wide.

Standards of Professional Practice

American Nurses Association (ANA, 2010c) explains the role of autonomy in nursing practice:

> All nursing practice, regardless of specialty, role, or setting, is fundamentally independent practice. Registered nurses are accountable for nursing judgments made and actions taken in the course of their nursing practice, therefore, the registered nurse is responsible for assessing individual competence and is committed to the process of lifelong learning. Registered nurses develop and maintain current knowledge and skill through formal and continuing education and seek certification when it is available in their areas of practice (p. 24, para. 2)

In order for nurses to acquire a fully autonomous practice, one must subscribe to lifelong learning to maintain and develop one's knowledge. Nurses are unable to make accurate and timely independent decisions without meeting the competencies of Standard 12: Education, such as:

- "Participates in ongoing educational activities related to nursing and interprofessional knowledge bases and professional topics"
- "Demonstrates a commitment to lifelong learning through self-reflection and inquiry for learning and personal growth" (ANA, 2015c, p. 76)

In addition to improving quality, hospitals must also improve patients' perceptions of their hospital experience. Patients' perception of care, known as patient satisfaction, is tied to hospital reimbursement from Medicare through the Hospital Consumer Assessment of Healthcare Providers and Services (HCAHPS) scores (Agency for Healthcare Research and Quality, 2017). Patients receive a HCAHPS survey about their hospital experience in the mail after discharge.

Due to potential implications of reduced reimbursement, nurses and the entire healthcare system must focus care on practices that positively impact the patient experience. The list below shares some of the HCAHPS topics where nurses are can positively impact the patient experience through autonomous practice:

- Communication with nurses
- Responsiveness of hospital staff
- Pain management
- Communication about medication
- Discharge information
- Cleanliness of the hospital environment
- Quietness of the hospital environment (Centers for Medicare and Medicaid [CMS], 2019)

Depending on the work setting, nurses may not have decision-making authority in all aspects of care. Authority to make certain patient care decisions depends on allowances made by the employer (Rau, Kumar, & McHugh, 2017). For example, a nurse may want to make an independent decision about an intravenous catheter, though the employer may have processes in place that overrule the nurse's decision. Often times such processes are in place to improve quality.

The ANA (n. d.-c) created the Magnet Recognition Program for healthcare organizations who strive for nursing excellence. The program designates Magnet Recognition to organizations worldwide whose nurse leaders have successfully transformed their nursing goals to improve patient outcomes. Magnet Recognition offers nurses education and professional development, leading to greater autonomy in nursing practice. The ANA (n. d.-c) has identified 14 characteristics of Magnet Recognition, known as Forces of Magnetism. Force 9 is Autonomy, which reads:

> Autonomous nursing care is the ability of a nurse to assess and provide nursing actions as appropriate for patient care based on competence, professional expertise and knowledge. The nurse is expected to practice autonomously, consistent with professional standards. Independent judgment is expected within the context of interdisciplinary and multidisciplinary approaches to patient/resident/client care (ANA, n. d.-c, para. 11).

Autonomy is an essential characteristic of the nursing profession; therefore, it is imperative nurses understand the importance of autonomy, and the factors that enhance or reduce autonomy in one's practice. The ability to make independent decisions about care has a multitude of benefits on health outcomes, the patient experience, financial reimbursement, job satisfaction, and the health and well-being of the nurse. These topics are discussed below.

Benefits of Nursing Autonomy

Since nurses represent the largest percentage of healthcare providers, they play an important role in transforming healthcare. When nurses make autonomous decisions about care, they are questioning the status quo, they are looking to find ways to improve the healthcare system, improve health outcomes, reduce adverse events, improve patient satisfaction, and quality. While providing quality care has always been paramount, quality of care is under particular scrutiny in the current healthcare system. Hospitals and healthcare providers are expected to deliver patient-centered and value-based care (Rau et al., 2017), otherwise healthcare organizations are negatively impacted with financial penalties (CMS, 2018).

Rau et al. (2017) studied nurse autonomy and its impact on quality of care and 30-day mortality rates. Research found hospitals with higher levels of nurse autonomy had reduced 30-day mortality rates. Another study (Maurits, Veer, Groenewegen, & Francke, 2017) found higher rates of autonomy in the home care setting led to improved job satisfaction for BSN prepared nurses. The following is a summary of the benefits of autonomous nursing practice:

- Sense of professional satisfaction by developing quality, responsive, and humanized care, essential for patient survival (Weston, 2008)
- Job satisfaction (Weston, 2008)
- Feelings of pleasure and appreciation of providing care (Weston, 2008)
- Reduced 30-day mortality rates (Rau et al., 2017)
- Enhanced job satisfaction (Weston, 2008)
- Improved quality of nursing performance (Weston, 2008)

Impact of Low Levels of Nurse Autonomy

The lack of nursing autonomy negatively impacts nurses, patients, other members of the team and the organization as a whole. When nurses do not have the freedom to use their knowledge and skills to provide care, nurses can suffer from physical and psychological harm, eventually leading to reduce quality of care, and ultimately reduced reimbursement. Papathanassoglou et al. (2012) shares the following adverse effects of low levels of nursing autonomy:

- Lack of motivation
- Physical illness
- Moral distress
- Depersonalization
- Professional and personal devaluation
- Depression

Papathanassoglou et al. (2012) studied how autonomy impacted nurses' level of moral distress and collaboration with physicians. The study found nurses with lower levels of autonomy had higher rates of moral distress and lower levels of nurse-physician collaboration. Nurses who inconsistently made independent decisions collaborated less often, which puts patients at risk for poorer quality of care. If providers do not collaborate with nurses, they are missing important information about patient needs and vital nursing insight. Sollami, Caricati, and Sarli (2015) found teamwork and nurse-physician collaboration improved quality of care, decreased work conflicts, and improved team motivation. The lack of collaboration will eventually lead to poorer outcomes and quality care.

Level of autonomy and collaboration with physicians must be evaluated when quality of care, nurse distress, and poor team motivation are present. Nurses must make efforts to identify how team processes and policies impact autonomy and collaboration. The following section reviews factors that enhance and inhibit autonomy.

Factors Known to Enhance Autonomy

Strapazzon Bonfada, Pinno, and Camponogara (2018) found the following factors enhanced nurses' autonomy in the hospital setting:

- Effective communication with members of the interdisciplinary team
- Positive interpersonal relationships with coworkers
- Organization and documentation of patient care
- Technical and scientific knowledge
- Leadership
- Cultural knowledge
- Professional experience
- Professional appreciation
- Policies that support autonomous decision-making

Specialty certification offers nurses an advanced knowledge base and enhanced competencies, skills, and qualifications. Nurses who have earned a certification benefits from enhanced autonomy in practice, empowerment, higher level of professionalism and improved interdisciplinary collaboration (Fritter & Shimp, 2016).

Skår (2009) found nurses who established a relationship with their patients led to a better understanding of the patient's situation. Nurses were better positioned to advocate for their patient's needs. As a result, Skår (2009) found a stronger nurse-patient relationship gave nurses the opportunity to provide holistic care and act autonomously.

Factors Known to Inhibit Autonomy

- Lack of technical-scientific knowledge
- Hierarchy
- Authoritarian leadership (oppressive, domineering)
- Physical and emotional exhaustion (work overload)
- Negative working conditions (bureaucracy, compliance with regulations, hierarchy)
- Lack of human (i.e. nurses/nursing shortage) and material resources
- Lack of communication with managers (Strapazzon Bonfada et al., 2018)

Skår (2009) found nurses who had a lack of control over their environment had restricted autonomy. For example, charge nurses with limited decision-making power and inability to confer with the physician or other nurses struggled to make autonomous decisions. These are examples of where nurses need evaluate their work environment and create a plan on how to gain more control over their practice. Nurses can take it upon themselves to create ways to empower the charge nurse role, suggest innovative processes for communication with the team. Exploring ways to transform the work environment to one that values communication and collaboration is an essential step towards autonomous practice.

Strategies to Improve Autonomy

As previously discussed, knowledge and confidence are the two key factors to autonomous practice. Actions taken to advance knowledge and confidence will lead to improving a nurse's ability to make independent decisions about clinical practice. Keep in mind that nurses may have the personal ability (knowledge and confidence) to make autonomous decisions, though it does not mean such decisions can be made. Nurses must continually evaluate their work setting and environment to ensure they have the freedom to make independent decisions. Investigating policies and processes that restrain nursing autonomy is an essential step for improving autonomy (control over one's practice).

Level of nursing autonomy is largely influenced by the relationship with medical providers. Autonomy can be negatively impacted when nurses have no recourse or input about patient care, or they are completely reliant on the doctor to perform care. Establishing a professional and collegial relationship with providers is an important step in gaining their trust and respect. Nurses need to be assertive and advocate for their patients by offering the provider and the team ideas, relevant literature, and professional insight on best practices.

Another way nurses can improve their knowledge and develop skills and competencies is through participation in professional nursing organizations. Membership offers nurses a multitude of educational opportunities:

- Specialty certification
- Networking
- Mentoring
- Peer-reviewed journal subscriptions
- Continuing education modules, webinars
- Discounts on attending conferences

Involvement in scientific and nursing-related conferences, and other healthcare forums, strengthens professional identity, thus allowing nurses to reach higher levels of autonomy in their practice (Roshanzadeh, Aghaei, Kashani, Pasaeimehr, & Tajabadi, 2018). A comprehensive review of the benefits of joining professional nursing organizations can be found in week 7 resources.

Shared governance is an organizational/decision-making model where managers share the power of decision-making on patient care issues with nurses (Church, Baker, & Berry, 2008). When nurses have the opportunity to share their opinions and ideas concerning decisions that impact patient care, this type of authority promotes nurses' autonomy (Hoying & Allen, 2011). Nurses are able to make more independent decisions as a result of having input on how care should be provided. See the chapter on *Nursing Accountability* for more information about shared governance.

Managers play a pivotal role in improving nurses' confidence by supporting and encouraging nurses to make autonomous decisions (Roshanzadeh et al., 2018). In order to support nurses, managers must examine unit and hospital policies that support nursing autonomy and create opportunities to reinforce nurse-physician collaboration. Actions that bring team members together to share knowledge and expertise with each other support a patient-centered care focus.

Nurses have been chosen number one for the most honest and ethical profession for many years (Brenan, 2017). Maintaining this positive public image is essential for a strong professional identity and movement towards a more autonomous practice (Strapazzon Bonfada et al., 2018). Nurses can advocate for a more autonomous profession by seeking out more influential positions within healthcare organizations. Papathanassoglou et al. (2012) discusses how expanding professional nursing roles can improve autonomy by giving nurses more decision-making power. In order to expand roles, nurses need to reflect on their career goals and create a personal nursing philosophy and a professional development plan. See Week 2 resources for a comprehensive review of career goals and planning.

Considering all the members of the healthcare team, nurses spend the most time with patients. Nurses know their patients and family well, learning about their needs, wants, and goals. Consequently, nurses are eager to advocate for their patients, and want to make decisions they know will meet their patient's goals and lead to positive outcomes. When nurses work in an environment where they can make independent decisions based on patient needs, everyone benefits. Nurses meet their goals of providing patient- and family-centered care, and the patient receives the safe, quality care they deserve.

In order to transform the delivery of care, nurses must exercise their autonomy. It's through autonomous practice that nurses are able to use their critical thinking skills, experience, and specialized knowledge to provide exceptional nursing care.

References

Altmann, T. K. (2011). Registered nurses returning to school for a bachelor's degree in nursing: Issues emerging from a meta-analysis of the research. *Contemporary Nurse: A Journal for the Australian Nursing Profession, 39*(2), 256-272. http://doi.org/10.5172/conu.2011.256

Alvarado, S. E. (2019). The indelible weight of place: Childhood neighborhood disadvantage, timing of exposure, and obesity across adulthood. *Health and Place, 58*, 1-48. http://doi.org/10.1016/j.healthplace.2019.102159

American Association of Colleges of Nursing. (n.d.). *Academic progression in nursing: moving together toward a highly educated nursing workforce*. https://www.aacnnursing.org/News-Information/Position-Statements-White-Papers/Academic-Progression-in-Nursing

American Association of Colleges of Nursing. (2005). *Joint statement on delegation*. https://www.ncsbn.org/Delegation_joint_statement_NCSBN-ANA.pdf

American Association of Colleges of Nursing. (2008, October 20). *The essentials of baccalaureate education for professional nursing practice*. https://www.aacnnursing.org/Portals/42/Publications/BaccEssentials08.pdf

American Association of Colleges of Nursing. (2000, December 12). *The baccalaureate degree in nursing as minimal preparation for professional practice*. https://www.aacnnursing.org/News-Information/Position-Statements-White-Papers/Bacc-Degree-Prep

American Association of Colleges of Nursing. (2020a, April). *The impact of education on nursing practice*. https://www.aacnnursing.org/News-Information/Fact-Sheets/Impact-of-Education

American Association of Colleges of Nursing. (2020b). *Who we are*. http://www.aacnnursing.org/About-AACN

American Nurses Association. (n. d.-a). *About ANA*. https://www.nursingworld.org/ana/about-ana/

American Nurses Association. (n. d.-b). *About pathway*. https://www.nursingworld.org/organizational-programs/pathway/overview/

American Nurses Association. (1965). American Nurses' Association's first position on education for nursing. *The American Journal of Nursing, 65*(12), 106-111. https://www.jstor.org/stable/3419707

American Nurses Association. (1980). *Nursing: A social policy statement*. Kansas City, MO: Author.

American Nurses Association. (2012, June). *The value of nursing care coordination: A white paper of the American Nurses Association*. https://www.nursingworld.org/~4afc0d/globalassets/practiceandpolicy/health-policy/care-coordination-white-paper-3.pdf

American Nurses Association. (2014, November 12). *ANA position statement: Profession role competence*. https://www.nursingworld.org/practice-policy/nursing-excellence/official-position-statements/id/professional-role-competence/

American Nurses Association. (2015a). *Guide to the code of ethics for nurses with interpretive statements* (2nd ed.). Author.

American Nurses Association. (2015b). *Guide to nursing's social policy statement. Understanding the profession from social contract to social covenant*. Author.

American Nurses Association. (2015c). *Scope and standards of practice* (3rd ed.). Author.

American Nurses Association. (2019, April 1). *Joint statement on delegation*. https://www.nursingworld.org/~4962ca/ globalassets/practiceandpolicy/nursing-excellence/ana-position-statements/nursing-practice/ana-ncsbn-joint-statement-on-delegation.pdf

Anthony, M. K. (2004). Shared governance models: The theory, practice, and evidence. *Online Journal of Issues in Nursing, 9*(1), 1-13. https://ojin.nursingworld.org/MainMenuCategories/ANAMarketplace/ANAPeriodicals/OJIN/TableofContents/ Volume92004/No1Jan04/SharedGovernanceModels.aspx

Association of Community College Trustees. (2017, December 14). *Joint statement on the baccalaureate degree as entry-level preparation for professional nursing practice*. https://www.acct.org/article/joint-statement-baccalaureate-degree-entry-level-preparation-professional-nursing-practice

Battié, R., & Steelman, V. M. (2016). Accountability in nursing practice: Why it is important for patient safety. *ACORN: The Journal of Perioperative Nursing in Australia, 29*(4), 11–14. http://doi.org/10.1016/j.aorn.2014.08.008

Blais, K.K., & Hayes, J.S. (2011). *Professional nursing practice: Concepts and perspectives*. (6th ed.). Pearson Education, Inc.

Brown, J. (1992). *The definition of a profession: The authority of metaphor in the history of intelligence testing, 1890-1930*. Princeton University Press.

Bruce, J. C. (2018). Nursing in the 21st Century. Challenging its values and roles. *Professional Nursing Today, 22*(1), 44–48. http://www.pntonline.co.za/index.php/PNT

Buhai, S. L. (2012). Profession: A definition. *Fordham Urban Law Journal, 40*(1), 242-273. https://ir.lawnet.fordham.edu/ulj/all_issues.html

Centers for Disease Control and Prevention. (2003, February 13). Public health and aging: Trends in aging-United States and worldwide. *MMWR Weekly 52*(6), 101-106. https://www.cdc.gov/mmwr/preview/mmwrhtml/mm5206a2.htm

Centers for Disease Control and Prevention. (2018a, July 18). *Arthritis-related statistics*. https://www.cdc.gov/arthritis/data_statistics/arthritis-related-stats.htm

Centers for Disease Control and Prevention. (2018b, November 8). *Leading indicators for chronic diseases and risk factors*. https://chronicdata.cdc.govmaps/index.html

Centers for Disease Control and Prevention. (2018c, January 18). *Smoking is down, but almost 38 million American adults still smoke*. https://www.cdc.gov/media/releases/2018/p0118-smoking-rates-declining.html

Centers for Disease Control and Prevention. (2019, December 2). *Heart disease*. https://www.cdc.gov/nchs/fastats/heart-disease.htm

Centers for Disease Control and Prevention. (2020a, April 22) *National Center for Chronic Disease Prevention and Health Promotion, Division of Nutrition, Physical Activity, and Obesity. Data, Trend and Maps*. https://www.cdc.gov/nccdphp/dnpao/data-trends

Centers for Disease Control and Prevention. (2020b). *National diabetes statistics report, 2020 estimates of diabetes and its burden in the United States*. https://www.cdc.gov/diabetes/pdfs/data/statistics/national-diabetes-statistics-report.pdf

Centers for Disease Control and Prevention. (2020c). *Percent of adults aged 18 and older who have obesity, National*. https://chronicdata.cdc.gov/Nutrition-Physical-Activity-and-Obesity/Percent-of-adults-aged-18-and-older-who-have-obesi/tv7q-8s5b

Centers for Medicare and Medicaid. (2019). *CAHPS adult hospital survey*. https://www.hcahpsonline.org/en/

Church, J.A., Baker, P. & Berry, D.M. (2008). Shared governance: A journey with continual mile markers. *Nursing Management, 39*(4), 34-40. http://doi.org/10.1097/01.NUMA.0000316058.20070.8c

Colby, S. L., & Ortman, J. M. (2015, March). *Projections of the size and composition of the US population: 2014 to 2060: Population estimates and projections.* https://www.census.gov//content/dam/Census/library/publications/2015/demo/p25-1143.pdf

Cox, S., & Beeson, G. (2018). Getting accountability right. *Nursing Management, 49*(9), 24–30. http://doi.org/10.1097/01.NUMA.0000544458.73828.42

Donabedian, A. (1976). Forward, in M. Phaneuf, *The nursing audit: Self-regulation in nursing* practice (2nd ed.). Appleton-Century-Crofts.

Donley, R., & Flaherty, M. J. (2002). Revisiting the American Nurses Association's first position on education for nurses. *Online Journal of Issues in Nursing, 7*(2), 1-17. https://www.researchgate.net/profile/Rosemary_Donley/publication/11315533_Revisiting_the_American_Nurses_Association's_First_Position_on_Education_for_Nurses/links/564c916b08ae020ae9fabcd7.pdf

Fritter, E., & Shimp, K. (2016). What does certification in professional nursing practice mean? *MedSurg Nursing, 25*(2), 131-132. https://go.gale.com/ps/anonymous?id=GALE%7CA452585842&sid=googleScholar&v=2.1&it=r&linkaccess=fulltext&issn=10920811&p=AONE&sw=w

Golanowski, M., Beaudry, D., Kurz, L., Laffey, W. J., & Hook, M. L. (2007). Interdisciplinary shared decision-making: Taking shared governance to the next level. *Nursing Administration Quarterly, 31*(4), 341-353. http://doi.org/10.1097/01.NAQ.0000290431.72184.5a

Gormley K. J. (1996). Altruism: A framework for caring and providing care. *International Journal of Nursing Studies, 33*(6), 581–588. https://doi.org/10.1016/S0020-7489(96)00013-2

Health Resources and Services Administration. (2010, September). *The registered nurse population: Findings from the 2008 national sample survey of registered nurses.* https://bhw.hrsa.gov/sites/default/files/bhw/nchwa/rnsurveyfinal.pdf

Hess, R. G. Jr. (2004). From bedside to boardroom: Nursing shared governance. *Online Journal of Issues in Nursing, 9*(1), 1-10. http://ojin.nursingworld.org/MainMenuCategories/ANAMarketplace/ANAPeriodicals/OJIN/TableofContents/Volume92004/No1Jan04/FromBedsidetoBoardroom.html

Hoying, C., & Allen, S. R. (2011). Enhancing shared governance for interdisciplinary practice. *Nursing Administration Quarterly, 35*(3), 252-259. http://doi.org/10.1097/NAQ.0b013e3181ff3a1d

Huston, C. (2013). The impact of emerging technology on nursing care: Warp speed ahead. *The Online Journal of Issues in Nursing, 18*(2). http://doi.org/10.3912/OJIN.Vol18No02Man01

Institute of Medicine. (2011). *The future of nursing: Leading change advancing health.* National Academies Press

Joel, L. A., & Kelly, L. (2002). *The nursing experience: Trends, challenges, and transitions.* McGraw-Hill.

Jones-Schenk, J., Leafman, J., Wallace, L., & Allen, P. (2017). Addressing the cost, value, and student debt in nursing education. *Nursing Economics, 35*(1), 7-13. https://www.nursingeconomics.net/necfiles/2017/JF17/7.pdf

Krugman, M. & Goode, J. C. (2018). BSN preparation for RNs: The time is now! *The Journal of Nursing Administration, 48*(2), 57–60. http://doi.org/10.1097/NNA.0000000000000572

Lee, V., Reilly, R., Laux, K., & Robitaille, A. (2018). Compassion, connection, community: Preserving traditional core values to meet future challenges in oncology nursing practice. *Canadian Oncology Nursing Journal, 28*(3), 212-216. http://www.canadianoncologynursingjournal.com/index.php/conj/article/view/914

Manthey, M. (2018). Substance use disorders and the American Nurses Association Code of Ethics for Nurses. *Creative Nursing, 24*(3), 163–165. http://doi.org/10.1891/1946-6560.24.3.163

Massachusetts Department of Higher Education Nursing. (2016, March). *Massachusetts nurse of the future nursing core competencies: Registered nurse.* http://www.mass.edu/nahi/documents/NOFRNCompetencies_updated_March2016.pdf

Maurits, E. E., Veer, A. J., Groenewegen, P. P., & Francke, A. L. (2017). Home-care nursing staff in self-directed teams are more satisfied with their job and feel they have more autonomy over patient care: A nationwide survey. *Journal of Advanced Nursing,* (10), 2430-2441. http://doi.org/10.1111/jan.13298

McNeil, B. J., Elfrink, V., Beyea, S. C., Pierce, S. T., & Bickford, C. J. (2006). Computer literacy study: Report of qualitative findings. *Journal of Professional Nursing, 22*(1), 52-59. http://doi.org/10.1016/j.profnurs.2005.12.006

Miller, J. G. (2012). *QBQ!: The question behind the question: Practicing personal accountability at work and in life.* Penguin Random House

National Academy of Sciences. (2020). *About us.* http://www.nationalacademies.org/hmd/About-HMD.aspx

National Council of State Boards of Nursing. (2019a 2020a). *About U.S. nursing regulatory bodies.* https://www.ncsbn.org/about-boards-of-nursing.htm

National Council of State Boards of Nursing. (2020b). *Explore NCSBN through the years.* https://timeline.ncsbn.org/index.htm

National Council of State Boards of Nursing. (2020c). *History.* https://www.ncsbn.org/history.htm

National Institute of Nursing Research. (n.d.). *Mission & strategic plan.* https://www.ninr.nih.gov/aboutninr/ninr-mission-and-strategic-plan

National League for Nursing. (2020). *Overview.* http://www.nln.org/about/overview

Near, J. P., & Miceli, M. P. (1985). Organizational dissidence: The case of whistle-blowing. *Journal of Business Ethics, 4*(1), 1–16. http://doi.org/10.1007/BF00382668

New York State Senate. (2017). *Senate bill S6768.* https://www.nysenate.gov/legislation/bills/2017/s6768

Oreofe, A. I., & Oyenike, A. M. (2018). Transforming practice through nursing innovative patient centered care: Standardized nursing languages. *International Journal of Caring Sciences, 11*(2), 1319–1322. https://www.internationaljournalofcaringsciences.org/docs/76_oyenike_special_10_5.pdf

Papathanassoglou, E., Karanikola, M., Kalafati, M., Giannakopoulou, M., Lemonidou, C., & Albarran J. (2012). Professional autonomy, collaboration with physicians, and moral distress among European intensive care nurses. *American Journal of Critical Care, 21*(2), 41-52. http://doi.org/10.4037/ajcc2012205

Pirschel, C. (2017, April 3). Competencies create expert, accountable nurses delivering quality care. *ONS Voice, 32*(4), 12-16. https://voice.ons.org/news-and-views/core-competencies-of-oncology-nurses

Rao, A. D., Kumar, A., & McHugh, M. (2017). Better nurse autonomy decreases the odds of 30-day mortality and failure to rescue. *Journal of Nursing Scholarship, 49*(1), 73-79. http://doi.org/10.1111/jnu.12267

Reinhart, R. J. (2020, January 6). Nurses continue to rate highest in honesty, ethics. Gallup. https://news.gallup.com/poll/274673/nurses-continue-rate-highest-honesty-ethics.aspx

Ritchie, L., & Gilmore, C. (2013). What does it mean to be a professional nurse? *Kai Tiaki Nursing New Zealand, 19*(8), 32.

Strategies of Professional Nursing Autonomy by Mostafa Roshanzadeh, Mirhossein Aghaei, Ehsan Kashani, Zahra Pasaeimehr, and Ali Tajabadi is licensed under Creative Commons Attribution CC BY-SA 4.0 International License.

Salmond, S. W., & Echevarria, M. (2017). Healthcare transformation and changing roles for nursing. *Orthopedic nursing, 36*(1), 12. http://doi.org/10.1097/NOR.0000000000000308

Skår, R. (2009). The meaning of autonomy in nursing practice. *Journal of Clinical Nursing, 19*(15-16), 2226-2234. http://doi.org/10.1111/j.1365-2702.2009.02804.x

Smiley, R. A., Lauer, P., Bienemy, C., Berg, J. G., Shireman, E., Reneau, K. A., & Alexander, M. (2018). The 2017 national nursing workforce survey. *Journal of Nursing Regulation, 9*(3), S1-S88. https://doi.org/10.1016/S2155-8256(18)30131-5

Sollami, A., Caricati, L., & Sarli, L. (2015). Nurse–physician collaboration: A meta-analytical investigation of survey scores. *Journal of Interprofessional Care, 29*(3), 223-229. http://doi.org/10.3109/13561820.2014.955912

Statewide Peer Assistance for Nurses. (2018). *About us.* https://www.statewidepeerassistance.org

Strapazzon Bonfada, M., Pinno, C., & Camponogara, S. (2018). Potentialities and limits of nursing autonomy in a hospital environment. *Journal of Nursing UFPE, 12*(8), 2235-2246. http://doi.org/10.5205/1981-8963-v12i8a234915p2235-2246-2018

Thomas, C. M., & Siela, D. (2011, April 11). The impaired nurse: Would you know what to do if you suspected substance abuse? *American Nurse Today, 6*(8). https://www.myamericannurse.com/the-impaired-nurse-would-you-know-what-to-do-if-you-suspected-substance-abuse/

Traynor, M., Boland, M., & Buus, N. (2010). Autonomy, evidence and intuition: Nurses and decision-making. *Journal of Advanced Nursing, 66*(7), *1584-1591.* http://doi.org/10.1111/j.1365-2648.2010.05317

Thomas, C. M., McIntosh, C. E., Sigma Theta Tau, I., & Mensik, J. (2016). *A Nurse's step-by-step guide to transitioning to the professional nurse role.* Sigma Theta Tau International.

Thorne, S., Kuo, M., Armstrong, E-A., McPherson, G., Harris, S.R., & Hislop, T.G. (2005). "Being Known": Patients' perspectives of the dynamics of human connection in cancer care. *Psycho-Oncology, 14,* 887–898. http://doi.org/10.1002/pon.945

U.S. Department of Health and Human Services. (2020, May 19). *Social determinants of health.* https://www.healthypeople.gov/2020/topics-objectives/topic/social-determinants-of-health

Watson, J. (1981). Nursing's scientific quest. *Nursing Outlook, 29*(7), 413-16.

Watson, J. (1988). *Nursing: Human science and human care: A theory of nursing.* Jones and Bartlett.

Watson, J. (2008). *Human caring science: A theory of nursing* (2nd ed.). Jones and Bartlett Learning.

Weber, E. (2017, September 26). What to do when a colleague is impaired. *American Nurse Today, 12*(9). https://www.myamericannurse.com/colleague-impaired/

Weston, M. J. (2008). Defining control over nursing practice and autonomy. *Journal of Nursing Administration, 38,* 404–408. http://doi.org/10.1097/01.NNA.0000323960.29544.e5

CHAPTER 2

Nursing Philosophy

Creating a personal nursing philosophy is akin to a journey of self-discovery. A nursing philosophy is a reflection of a personal and professional value system, beliefs, goals, ethics and one's relationship to the world at large. A philosophy may explain one's mission in life, or the impetus that led them to entering the nursing profession.

Creating a nursing philosophy helps nurses understand themselves better, recognize how thinking impacts actions, how goals are viewed, and how decisions are made throughout one's career. A nursing philosophy allows individuals to apply knowledge to its fullest extent, which leads to further nursing knowledge, and for some nurses, the inspiration to create theories (Marchuk, 2014).

Nursing Metaparadigm

Creating a nursing philosophy requires an understanding of the nursing metaparadigm. Hardy (1978) introduced the use of paradigms to nursing to share a comprehensive description of the profession. The nursing metaparadigm is the foundation for nursing knowledge and philosophy (Fawcett, 1984) and its four concepts, listed below, represent the core elements of all nursing theories.

- **Person:** recipient of nursing care
- **Nursing:** delivery of care, practice (goals, roles, and functions)
- **Environment:** surroundings of the patient (internal and external influences, physical and social)
- **Health:** level of wellness, well-being (Fawcett, 2005)

The four metaparadigm concepts interact and interrelate with each other. When creating one's nursing philosophy, individuals should consider how each of these concepts interrelate with the science and art of nursing, and how this connection applies to one's personal value and belief system.

Carper's (1978) seminal work on the *Fundamental Patterns of Knowing in Nursing* also assist nurses with creating a nursing philosophy. The four patterns of knowing are as follows:

- **Personal knowledge**
- **Empirics:** science of nursing
- **Ethics:** morality
- **Aesthetics:** art of nursing

Carper (1978) states the patterns of knowing represent the complexity and diversity within nursing practice. Incorporating the patterns of knowing into one's philosophy symbolizes a personal perspective and significance for one's practice. The patterns of knowing are not exclusive of each other, similar to the metaparadigm, instead, the elements of each pattern work together to explain nursing practice as a whole.

Reflecting on the four patterns of knowing brings about awareness of personal and professional knowledge, moral and ethical beliefs, science (such as research and evidence-based practice), and a creative imagination (aesthetics). Carper (1978) summarizes the meaning of nursing within the framework of the four patterns of knowing:

> Nursing thus depends on the scientific knowledge of human behavior in health and in illness, the esthetic perception of significant human experiences, a personal understanding of the unique individuality of the self and the capacity to make choices within concrete situations involving particular moral judgments (p. 22).

Creating a Personal Philosophy

As nurses reflect on values, beliefs, patterns of knowing, and the metaparadigm, the following questions can be of assistance while creating a nursing philosophy:

- What is professional nursing and what does it mean to you?
- How is art represented in your practice?
- How does science impact your practice?
- What is health? What does it mean to you?
- What is the relationship between society and health?
- How does the Code of Ethics guide your practice?
- How do you view the recipient of your care?
- What is the role of nursing in society as a whole?
- How do your values and beliefs align with the Standards of Professional Practice?
- What is the meaning of life, both personally and professionally?

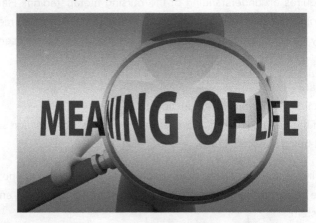

A nursing philosophy is dynamic, it will always be a work in progress. Nursing philosophies change throughout one's career due to new knowledge, and personal and professional experiences. As a philosophy changes, career aspirations may also change. Reading one's philosophy on a regular basis helps nurses recall a perspective from the past, which may inspire new desires and goals for the future.

Professional Development

A rapidly expanding and complex healthcare environment requires nurses with advanced knowledge, skills, and competencies to meet the growing demand for a highly skilled workforce. Nurses also need to bolster their existing practice to ensure progress and readiness for future challenges and maximum growth. Through professional development activities, nurses are able to reach their professional goals for growth and development, and at the same time meet the needs of a demanding healthcare environment. Creating a professional development plan (PDP) is an integral part of professional nursing practice, and planning should begin as early as possible in one's career.

Professional development includes activities such as specialty certification, additional degrees, attending conferences, publishing scholarly work, committee membership, and more. Planning one's professional development requires planning and goal setting. Contemplating a realistic timeline, financial resources, time management, and other considerations is a very important part of the plan.

Professional growth and development are an expectation set forth in the American Nurses Association (ANA, 2015c) Nursing Scope and Standards of Practice. Standard 12, Education, states "The registered nurse seeks knowledge and competence that reflects current nursing practice and promotes futuristic thinking" (p. 76). The Standard lists the competencies required by the registered nurse. The list below shares a few of the competencies for professional growth and development:

- Demonstrates a commitment to lifelong learning through self-reflection and inquiry for learning and personal growth.
- Identifies learning needs based on nursing knowledge and the various roles the nurse may assume.
- Facilitates a work environment supportive of ongoing education of healthcare professionals (ANA, 2015c, p. 76)

Professional development is an essential task for every nurse, whether the goal is to seek a new nursing role or to remain at a current position. Regardless of the long-term goal, PDPs are focused on enhancing one's career, planning for the future, paving the way towards a new job and career that meets your personal and professional goals. Creating PDPs gives nurses the momentum and excitement to reach new, stimulating opportunities, leading to a successful and satisfying career (Öznacar & Mümtazoğlu, 2017).

Evaluating a PDP on a regular basis gives nurses control over their practice, and ultimately, their future. Nurses have the power to free themselves from a job where their knowledge and skills may feel stagnant or there is no opportunity for advancement. A PDP offers nurses opportunities that build on strengths and passions, leading to a more gratifying and rewarding career.

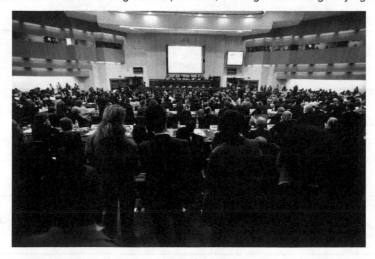

Professional Nursing Roles

The nursing profession offers a wide array of job opportunities. Nurses can choose to work in a variety of practice settings that fits one's goals. In order to keep current with the changing healthcare environment and achieve a satisfying nursing career, creating a PDP is key. See Table 1 for a brief list of professional nursing roles with education requirements and associated certifications.

Table 1 shares professional nursing roles with degree requirements and certifications

Table 1: Professional Nursing Roles

Nursing Roles	Minimum Education	Certifications
Diabetic Nurse Educator	BSN preferred	Certified Diabetes Educator (CDE)
Nurse Midwife	Masters	Certified Nurse-Midwife (CNM)
Pediatric Nurse	BSN preferred	Pediatric Nursing (RN-BC)
Forensic nurse	BSN preferred	Sexual Assault Nurse Examiner (SANE)
Medical/Surgical Nurse	BSN preferred	Medical/Surgical Nurse (RN-BC)
Nurse Anesthetist	Masters or DNP	Certified Registered Nurse Anesthetist (CRNA)
Wound Ostomy Continence Nurse	BSN preferred	Certified Wound Ostomy Continence Nurse (CWOCN) (different levels of WOCN cert.)
Case manager	BSN preferred	Nursing Case Management (RN-BC)
Clinical Nurse Specialist (choose setting)	Masters or DNP	Clinical Nurse Specialist (CNS-BS)
Hospice/Palliative Care Nurse	BSN preferred	Certified Hospice/Palliative Nurse (CHPN)
Nurse Educator (academic or clinical)	Masters, DNP or PhD	Certified Nurse Educator (CNE)
Director of Nursing	DNP or PhD	Nurse Executive Certification Advanced (NEA-BC)
Nurse Manager	BSN or Masters	Nurse Executive Certification (NE-BC)
School Nurse	BSN preferred	National Certified School Nurse (NCSN)
Psychiatric Mental Health Nurse Practitioner	Masters, DNP or PhD	Certified Psychiatric Mental Health Nurse Practitioner (PMHNP-BC)
BC = Board Certified		

Creating a Professional Development Plan

Creating a PDP takes time to reflect on one's life and experiences. The first step is to refer to one's personal nursing philosophy where values, inspirations, beliefs, reasons for entering the profession, and other ideas can be used to create goals. Reflecting on aspects of a workday that are pleasing or enjoyable also assist with creating goals for a PDP.

In addition, comprehensive research will need to be completed if interested in a specific nursing role. Researching a potential role will include learning about required education/certification, years of experience, cost of education, availability of scholarships and other funding opportunities, and more.

Consider the following questions while pondering career goals:

- What part of nursing practice inspires you?
- Why did you enter the nursing profession?
- Is there a particular work setting or specialty that you are drawn to?
- Are there activities in your current role that excite you?
- What are your strengths?
- Do you enjoy working with technology?
- Do you enjoy understanding how science and research impacts care?
- Do you enjoy teaching patients or coworkers?
- Are you interested in policy, improving practice for the profession as a whole?
- What elements of nursing practice are you are passionate about?

Chang (2000) writes about following one's passion, stating passion elicits feelings about the world being filled with possibilities. Passion is defined as "activities, ideas, and topics that elicit the emotions." (Chang, 2000, p. 19). Chang (2000) further defines passion as an intensity, a force that fuels our strongest emotions.

Think about activities of nursing practice that illicit passion, follow your heart when making decisions. Following one's passion helps find meaning in practice. Think back to the enthusiasm and feelings of excitement and fulfilled purpose that led to entering nursing school.

When nurses create their PDP by following their passions, the task becomes promising and positive, rather than overwhelming and frustrating. Creating a PDP requires time and thought, a process that cannot be rushed. Staying focused on the end goal of creating a future that melds with lifelong goals can overshadow any difficulties you may incur throughout the reflection, research, and planning phases.

Consider including some of the following activities in a PDP:

- Participate on a hospital committee
- Participate in shared governance in your unit
- Present updated evidence-based practice topic to unit staff monthly or quarterly
- Organize a unit committee based on a specific need
- Offer to be a mentor or preceptor for novice nurses on your unit
- Membership in professional organizations

Similar to a nursing philosophy, a PDP is dynamic and changes over time. Goals will be met at varying stages throughout one's career, and long-term career goals are bound to change as experience impacts knowledge and thinking. The desire to work on a medical/surgical unit now may be very different 10 years from now. Over time nurses learn more about themselves and their strengths and passions will inevitably change. The opportunities in nursing practice are endless, it's one of the countless benefits of working in this remarkable profession.

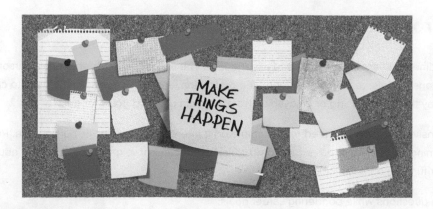

Benefits of Professional Development

Job Opportunities

Since the nursing profession offers multiple paths to licensure, nurses with varying types of degrees often compete with each other for certain nursing positions (acute care is one example). Depending on location, many employers require a baccalaureate degree (or working towards one) to be considered for hire. In addition, now that the BSN in 10 law has passed, current students entering nursing schools in NY will be required to earn a baccalaureate degree, adding more baccalaureate prepared nurses, and competition, into practice.

Creating a PDP with the job market and competition for nursing positions in mind, nurses can form a strategy for positions that may not have been available unless planning had been in place. Furthermore, nurses who include additional professional growth opportunities, such as certification or mentoring, in their PDP will be recognized for their added accomplishments.

Echevarria (2018) states membership in professional organizations helps nurses market themselves for future job opportunities. Sharing professional development activities on one's resume or curricula vitae (CV) demonstrates to potential employers the nurse's commitment to lifelong learning and advocacy for the professional. Participation in professional development opportunities meets competencies within Standard 8, Education, from the ANA (2015c) Nursing Scope and Standards of Practice stating, "Maintains professional portfolio that provides evidence of individual competence and lifelong learning" (p. 76).

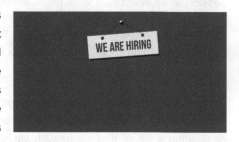

Recruiters seek out nurses who are actively seeking out professional development and often advertise job openings on professional organization sites. Depending on the organization, members may gain additional benefits with career development tools, such as writing a resume, mock interviews, and posting resumes to a job board (Echevarria, 2018).

Fulfilling Lifelong Learning Goals

Lifelong learning is an expectation of all nurses. Through professional development planning nurses can tailor learning activities to meet a variety of goals. Learning opportunities may be planned for license renewal or to meet a PDP goal. Planning a timeline to meet goals will ensure goals are met. Nurses need to be open to learning about an assortment of new knowledge, and accept constructive criticism (Mustafa, 2017). Continuing education on a variety of topics increases one's control over practice, ultimately leading to a satisfying job and career.

Mentoring

Mentoring unites colleagues together, helping each other grow professionally. Whether it's a novice nurse just entering the profession or an experienced nurse learning about a new specialty role, mentoring is an important way nurses can help each other with role transitions. Through mentoring, nurses are empowered by sharing their knowledge, which in turn strengthens the profession by securing competent practitioners and nurse leaders (Vance & Olsen, 1998). In addition, mentoring has been found to improve job satisfaction, and reduce the stress of working in a challenging environment (Jones, 2017).

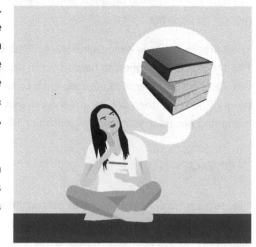

Mentoring helps nurses gain clinical knowledge and advice at a time when confidence and decision-making abilities are in the beginning stages. Nurses helping nurses is the foundation of professional practice. Some of the qualities and duties of mentors includes the following:

- Role model professional behaviors
- Offer career development advice
- Inspire others
- Encourage and support novice nurses
- Provide wisdom and share stories from their experience
- Trustworthy, confidants
- Mutual respect
- Open attitude

Mentoring activities meets the competencies within Standard 12, Leadership, from the ANA (2015c) Nursing Scope and Standards of Practice, stating, "The registered nurse leads within the professional practice setting and the profession" (p. 75). Mentoring may occur as a formal role, where a mentor and mentee have an official relationship or connection. Though nurses can mentor each other informally, by assisting others in need of advice and encouragement. The mentoring relationship is beneficial to both the mentor and the mentee, where both nurses benefitted from the process, stating they found their jobs more meaningful and satisfying (Malloy et al., 2015).

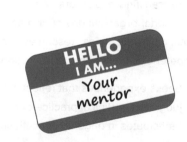

Healthcare organizations offer preceptors, mentoring, and residency programs for graduate nurses. Residency programs differ from other forms of mentoring or coaching where such programs offer organized educational sessions with assigned preceptors. Hospitals may create their own residency programs, though some private companies have created evidence-based residency programs used in healthcare organizations. For example, Vizient, a private organization, has teamed up with the American Association of Colleges of Nursing (AACN, 2019) and created a Nurse Residency program. Vizient's residency program, supported by The Joint Commission, the Institute of Medicine (IOM), and others, found participants had higher retention rates (93%) compared to the national average (83%) (AACN, 2019). Additionally, participants in the program led to achieving Magnet status in their workplace. For more information about the Nurse Residency program, visit the AACN website.

Nurse residency programs are essential for new nurses entering the healthcare field. The growth of residency programs is encouraging for nurses, employers, and ultimately, patient care. Establishing residency programs fulfills the third recommendation set forth by the IOM (2010) where healthcare organizations were tasked with supporting nurses to complete a transition-to-practice programs.

Professional organizations offer tools to help organizations create mentoring programs, such as the Academy of Medical-Surgical Nurses (AMSN). The AMSN offers guides tailored for mentors and mentees, and guidelines on how to create an environment where learning and sharing can occur. The mentorship program teaches nurse leaders how to match up mentors and mentees, tips for mentoring novice nurses, characteristics of successful mentoring, problems that may arise, how to evaluate the mentoring program, and more (Academy of Medical-Surgical Nurses, 2018). For more information about the AMSN mentoring program, visit the AMSN website.

The American Nurses Association (ANA, 2018) offers a mentoring program as a benefit of being a member of the organization. The program is designed to help new nurses acclimate to their new role and the nursing profession. The program is virtual, with mentors and mentees meeting each other online or via phone. The mentoring process begins with joining the mentoring program, then further details are shared with matching up a mentor to a mentee. For more information about the AMSN mentoring program, visit the ANA website.

Networking

Creating professional networks or connections with groups of healthcare professionals within and outside one's workplace helps nurses be cognizant of new career opportunities, advance quality patient care, and more (Sherman, 2018). Networking also offers nurses advice on how to overcome challenges and meet other nurses who have had similar experiences.

Professional networking assists nurses with developing relationships that offer professional growth and clinical knowledge to inform personal practice. Nurses who do not put forth the effort to network with peers and other healthcare professionals risk working in a silo, where care practices can become stagnant, risking the feeling of being in a "rut."

Sherman (2018) explains the benefits of networking for career opportunities, stating recruiters may not always advertise job openings, instead relying on referrals from professionals they work with, whose judgment they trust. Creating and sustaining a professional network is key to advancing your career and finding new opportunities.

Nurses can find a plethora of networking opportunities through national and specialty professional nursing organizations. Professional organizations offer many opportunities for professional growth, such as developing leadership skills, continuing education/certifications, resources for career development, and more (Echevarria, 2018). Networking meets the following competencies in Standard 8, Education, from the ANA (2015c) Nursing Scope and Standards of Practice:

- Seeks experiences that reflect current practice to maintain and advance knowledge, skills, abilities, attitudes, and judgment in clinical practice or role performance
- Participates in ongoing educational activities related to nursing and interprofessional knowledge bases and professional topics.
- Shares educational findings, experiences, and ideas with peers (ANA, 2015c, p. 76)

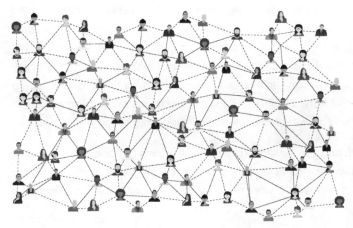

Planning short- and long-term goals helps nurses locate the most relevant, robust network of colleagues who can assist with seeking out new job opportunities. Many opportunities exist for networking within one's institution, such as presenting a new evidence-based practice at a unit meeting or volunteering for an institutional-wide committee.

Social media is another way to network with other healthcare professionals, such as Facebook, LinkedIn, and Twitter. Most professional organizations have their own Facebook and Twitter pages/feeds, making it easier for nurses to connect with other healthcare professionals that have similar interests and goals. Creating a LinkedIn account offers nurses opportunities to find mentors and colleagues who have similar interests as well.

While at a conference or other gatherings with healthcare professionals, Sherman (2018) encourages nurses to begin a conversation by asking any of the following questions:

- How did you get started in your role?
- What are your challenges?
- What significant changes are you seeing in your environment?
- What's the most innovative thing that's happening in your organization?
- What do you think will happen with healthcare reform?
- What trends do you see happening in nursing today?
- What advice would you give to an emerging nurse leader?
- How can I help you?
- Who else at this meeting would be helpful for me to speak with?

Sherman (2018) offers some additional advice about networking:

- Networking is about planning, developing the relationship over time. Do not inquire about a job too quickly.
- Build a community of colleagues, think about what you can do for others first. Volunteer to offer your assistance with setting up for a conference or sharing an article on a clinical procedure.
- Having an up-to-date LinkedIn page is essential, including a professional email address, outgoing phone message, and business cards. Always carry your business cards with you.
- Prepare for networking opportunities. Think about (and write down) topics to discuss or introductory questions.
- Be excited, and positive, to those you network with. Refrain from complaining about anything. Stay focused on building relationships.
- Relationship building begins with listening. Ask other people about themselves and their careers. Offer your ideas and ask questions, though be sure your personal dialog does not take up the entire conversation.
- Follow up with new relationships, whether it's sending a thank-you note or responding promptly to a request.
- Cultivate new relationships. Networking is an ongoing investment in professional development.

References

American Nurses Association. (2015c). *Scope and standards of practice* (3rd ed.). Author.

Association of Colleges of Nursing. (2019, March 25). *Vizient/AACN Nurse Residency Program*. https://www.aacnnursing.org/Portals/42/AcademicNursing/NRP/Nurse-Residency-Program.pdf

Academy of Medical-Surgical Nurses, 2020). *Mentoring*. https://www.amsn.org/professional-development/mentoring

Carper, B. A. (1978). Fundamental patterns of knowing in nursing. *Advances in Nursing Science, 1,* 13-23.

Chang, R. (2000). *The passion plan*. Jossey-Bass.

Fawcett, J. (1984). The metaparadigm of nursing: Present status and future refinements. *Journal of Nursing Scholarship, 16*(3), 84-87, http://doi.org/10.1111/j.1547-5069.1984.tb01393.x

Fawcett, J. (2005). *Contemporary nursing knowledge: Analysis and evaluation of nursing models and theories* (2nd ed.). F. A. Davis.

Hardy, M. E. (1978). Perspectives on nursing theory. *Advances in Nursing Science, 1,* 37-48.

Jones, S. J. (2017). Establishing a Nurse mentor program to improve nurse satisfaction and intent to stay. *Journal for Nurses in Professional Development*, (2), 76. http://doi.org/10.1097/NND.0000000000000335

Malloy, D. C., Fahey-McCarthy, E., Masaaki M., Yongho L., Eunhee C., Eri H., & Hadjistavropoulos, T. (2015). Finding meaning in the work of nursing: An international study. *Online Journal of Issues in Nursing, 20*(3), 7. http://doi.org/10.3912/OJIN.Vol20No03PPT02

Marchuk, A. (2014). A personal nursing philosophy in practice. *Journal of Neonatal Nursing, 20*, 266–273. http://doi.org/10.1016/j.jnn.2014.06.004

Mustafa, S. (2017). Importance of career development for individuals and organizations. *International Journal of Social Sciences & Educational Studies, 4*(2), 144-148. http://doi.org/10.23918/ijsses.v4i2sip144

Öznacar, B., & Mümtazoğlu, K. (2017). Career planning and mentorship in health care education. *Eurasia Journal of Mathematics Science & Technology Education, 13*(8), 4513-4521. http://doi.org/10.12973/eurasia.2017.00944a

Sherman, R. O., & Cohn, T. M. (2018, March 6). Why your nursing networks matter: Networks help you advance your career, provide high-quality care, and support your colleagues. *American Nurse Today, 13*(3), 9. https://www.myamericannurse.com/nursing-networks-matter/

Vance, C., & Olson, R. K. (1998). *The mentor connection in nursing*. Springer Publishing Company.

CHAPTER 3

Interprofessional Communication

Effective communication within the interdisciplinary team is one of the hallmarks to providing safe, quality care. Communication between individuals, groups, and organizations will either lead to successful interactions with high outcomes, or miscommunication, leading to poor quality, errors, unsafe care, and sentinel events (unexpected death or injury) (The Joint Commission [TJC], 2010; Weller, Boyd, & Cumin, 2014). To ensure effective interprofessional communication throughout acute care settings, TJC (n.d.) surveyors evaluate hospitals for compliance with patient-centered communication standards. TJC (n.d.) offers

Delivery of healthcare is complex, requiring clear and timely communication between multiple disciplines. It has been well documented that miscommunication is the root cause of medication errors, poor quality, and reduced health outcomes (O'Daniel & Rosenstein, 2008; TJC, 2015).

The Joint Commission on Accreditation of Healthcare Organizations (JCAHO, 2005) explains how a patient may interact with 50 different employees during a 4-day hospital stay. The opportunity for miscommunication is vast, compelling healthcare institutions to develop tools and training programs to improve communication throughout the entire organization (Institute of Medicine, 2010). Holmes et al. (2015) found implementation of training programs and use of standardized tools and simulation has the potential to improve patient safety.

Positive communication is a critical ingredient found throughout the culture of an effective organization. Leadership practices that will positively influence the organization's culture must be clearly defined. This plan will lead to the support that will encourage employees to identify problems early and be motivated to explore solutions and assist with implementation.

Standards of Practice

Professional nursing practice requires communication be maintained at a highly effective level. Developing a trusting relationship with patients, advocating for their needs, providing patient-centered care, and ensuring safe, quality care are vital reasons why this is indispensable.

As discussed in Week 1, the Scope and Standards of Practice, developed by the American Nurses Association (ANA, 2015c), serves as a template for professional nursing practice for all registered nurses. Standard 9, Communication, states, "The registered nurse communicates effectively in all areas of practice." (ANA, 2015c, p. 71). The following is a summary of the competencies of the Communication standard:

- Assesses one's own communication skills and effectiveness.
- Demonstrates cultural empathy when communicating.
- Maintains communication with interprofessional team and others to facilitate safe transitions and continuity in care delivery.
- Assesses communication ability, health literacy, resources, and preferences of healthcare consumers to inform the interprofessional team and others.
- Demonstrates continuous improvement of communication skills.
- Uses communication styles and methods that demonstrate caring, respect, deep listening, authenticity, and trust (ANA, 2015c, p. 71).

In Week 4, Leadership in Nursing, the Healthy Work Environment Model (HWEM) (American Association of Critical Care Nurses [AACN], 2016) is introduced. The model was created to improve practice environments and nursing practice by implementing six evidence-based standards. These standards have been found to improve and maintain a healthy work environment. The first standard is *Skilled Communication*, defined as nurses should be as proficient in communication skills as they are in clinical skills.

Becoming proficient in communicating with others and understanding the barriers to having successful interactions with others is a necessity for all nurses. Unless nurses view communication skills as equally important as honing clinical skills, work environment and patient outcomes will decline.

See Week 4 for more information about the Healthy Work Environment standards.

Types of Communication

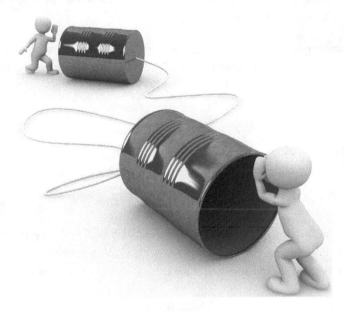

Communication is an interactive process whereby one person (the sender) influences another (the receiver) with information (a message). Messages are sent verbally, non-verbally, and by the tone of voice. Effective communication occurs when both the sender and receiver have a shared understanding of the message, and both perceive the message in the same way (JCAHO, 2005).

Verbal

- Verbal communication occurs through spoken language.

Paraverbal

- During verbal communication, the qualities of an individual's voice influence transmission of the message, including:
    - Tone: indicates a feeling, such as sadness, humor, anger
    - Inflection: rise and fall of the voice
    - Rhythm
    - Flow (O'Daniel & Rosenstein, 2008)

Non-Verbal

Non-verbal communication is an interactive process that occurs continuously, with and without verbal communication. Non-verbal behavior includes posture, body movements, mimics, facial expressions, gestures (O'Daniel & Rosenstein, 2008).Nurses can interpret their patient's body language and other non-verbal and paraverbal behaviors as part of the assessment process. Some patients may not have the ability to express themselves and body language may offer multiple inconclusive meanings. Proper follow up with additional questioning to confirm assumptions and understand new developments is prudent.

Benbenishty and Hannink (2015) states non-verbal communication has the capability to build trust by displaying an open body posture. In nursing, posture is a very important part of active listening during assessment or patient education. Consider body positions when listening to patient concerns, such as crossing arms or looking down at a patient during an interview. Positioning oneself and asking questions while looking at a laptop instead of looking directly at the patient with an open body posture will not foster open, effective, and honest communication.

Verbal communication has a smaller impact on the transmission of a message from one person to another and must be kept in perspective. Benbenishty and Hannink (2015) discuss the use of the 55/38/7 formula, used by communication psychologists, to understand the influence of each form of communication:

Verbal communication has a smaller impact on the transmission of a message from one person to another and must be kept in perspective. Communication psychologists refer to the 55/38/7 formula to understand the influence of each form of communication:

- **55%** non-verbal
- **38%** paraverbal
- **7%** verbal (Benbenishty & Hannink, 2015)

Non-Verbal Communication and Culture

The preferences and accepted norms for non-verbal behaviors listed below will vary depending on culture. Respecting patient preferences is essential for effective communication and developing trusting relationships with patients and team members. Nurses can empower patients by encouraging them to speak up if their preferences and values are overlooked or misunderstood.

- **Physical space:** Americans prefer more personal space, generally, than other cultures (*more information about physical space later in the chapter*)
- **Touching:** physical contact is associated with one's personality or communication style and can create discomfort. While touching an arm or shoulder shows support and empathy in American culture, it is best to ask patients if touching is okay.
- **Gestures:** some cultures become animated during communication, such as waving hands. Some cultures may find such gestures insulting and rude.
- **Eye contact:** in America, eye contact is understood as a sign of respect and a confident speaker. In contrast, eye contact can have negative connotations and can be insulting.
- **Silence:** some cultures are uncomfortable with silence, while others consider it as an opportunity to contemplate the message and meaning.
- **Body language:** verbal communication may be contradicted or confirmed by the use of body language. Consider the patient's impression when the nurse welcomes the patient to the unit with folded arms (Hosley & Molle, 2006; Leininger & McFarland, 2006).

Visit the online course to view the video on eye contact and non-verbal communication and the animation of miscommunication.

The sender and receiver take certain roles in the transmission of the message. The sender wants to be heard and receiver needs to share acknowledgement of the message. Transmission and acknowledgement may not occur for a number of reasons, including ineffective communication skills, conflicting non-verbal behaviors, or communication barriers. Evaluating one's communication behaviors and assessing for barriers is a constant challenge. Developing a broad base of communication skills is a necessity in a complex healthcare environment where communication is at the heart of interdisciplinary collaboration.

How does the nurse in charge of unlicensed staff at a group home, charge nurse at a hospital, or school nurse at an elementary school adapt the type of communication needed for their setting? They must evaluate the age/education level of receiver, common communication gaps and barriers, and through experience and seeking new solutions, gaps in communication can be reduced.

Communication Styles

It is undisputed that clear and accurate communication among the interdisciplinary team is vital for teamwork, collaboration, and ultimately, improved outcomes. Miscommunication is often the root cause reduced patient outcomes, often due to team members having diverse, and often conflicting communication styles. In order for teams to collaborate and share knowledge in a timely way, nurses need to understand their team members' communication styles. Recognizing and understanding team members' communication styles allows nurse to adjust their communication behaviors in order to reduce or prevent conflict and misunderstanding (Plonien, 2015).

In addition to learning about the three basic communication concepts (listed below), there are additional communication styles (Controller, Supporter, Promoter, and Analyzer) discussed at the Maximum Advantage website.

Communication Concepts

Passive Communication

- Not expressive
- Disregards their own rights, in turn encourages others to disregard their rights
- Speaks in an apologetic way
- Hesitant to share feelings with others
- Does not respond clearly
- Unconsciously accumulates complaints, which often causes an outburst, leading to unacceptable behavior and damaged relationships, in turn, causing blame and guilt, leading again to passive behavior (Tripathy, 2018)

Aggressive Communication

- Domineering
- Ambitious
- Demands others maintain order, especially when the situation gets out of control
- Bullies and intimidates peers (Tripathy, 2018)

Assertive Communication

- Considered the best form of communication, a balance between passive and aggressive
- Positive attitude
- Good listener, respects others' opinions
- Shares views in a calm and peaceful way
- Peers establish strong relationships with these communicators
- Expresses their thoughts, feelings, and emotions openly (Tripathy, 2018)

Omura, Maguire, Levett-Jones, and Stone (2016) discuss assertiveness as a powerful tool that eliminates the power differences between individuals. When individuals assert themselves, they are acting in their own best interest (such as advocating on the patient's behalf). Being assertive helps people stand up for themselves without feeling nervous or anxious.

Professional Communication

Professional communication is defined as the interaction between healthcare professionals with the principal goal of meeting health-related outcomes (Street & Mazor, 2017). When successful communication practices become a central component of an organization it can transform healthcare delivery. Successful nurse-patient interactions require a patient-centered approach, where patient preferences and values are the center of their communication. Nurses' communication skills and strategies need to be focused on educating, supporting, and empowering patients to manage their healthcare needs (Arnold and Boggs, 2019). Effective nurse-patient communication leads to patients having a better understanding of their health conditions leading them to be more active participants in their care.

Impact of Effective Communication:

- Development of nurse-physician relationships
- Increased patient satisfaction
- Early identification of changes in health status
- Improved understanding of patient's needs, health status
- Improved patient outcomes last longer (Arnold and Boggs, 2019)

Therapeutic Communication

Effective communication occurs when nurses establish trusting, therapeutic relationships with their patients (Arnold & Boggs, 2019). When nurses communicate in a therapeutic way, they are interacting for the purpose of learning about the patient's values, preferences, culture, interests, health needs, and developmental level (Rosenberg & Gallo-Silver, 2011). Developing therapeutic relationships is akin to Standard 1 (Assessment) of the Standards of Practice, where the nurse collects relevant information about the patient's health and condition. Knowledge of valuable patient information allows the nurse to create a patient-centered plan of care.

Peplau (1960), a well-known nursing theorist, states healthcare providers must be skilled in therapeutic communication. Effective therapeutic communication is a learned skill, requiring a concerted effort to acquire knowledge on essential communication skills. Peplau (1960) states nurses need to uphold the concept called *skilled mindfulness*, which is an approach that allows the healthcare provider to consider the unique needs of the patient and at the same time having a personal awareness of one's own responses and reactions. Peplau (1960) defines the nurse's role as the "participant observer."

Communication as an Art

Similar to nursing practice, effective communication is an art and a science. The art of communication is in the expression of how a message is conveyed. The speaker's personality, sense of humor, non-judgmental approach, level of respect, calmness, and their attitude towards the dialogue will vary between individuals (Arnold & Boggs, 2019). Reading the situation in which nurses communicate with patients, coworkers, and other healthcare professionals is also an important skill to master. The speaker needs to be intuitive to the receiver's preferences and needs, such as the amount of physical space, use of humor, or use of touch. Ensuring a positive first impression will influence the outcome of the interaction.

Communication Behaviors and Skills

The fundamental components of successful patient-centered communication include empathy, clarity, and honesty (Arnold & Boggs, 2019).

Empathy

Empathy is an essential component to building relationships with both patients and team members. Understanding each other's needs leads to better outcomes and improved work environments.

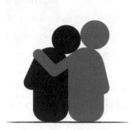

Empathy with Patients

Clinical empathy involves understanding patients' emotions and experiences regarding care. When nurses have empathy for a patient, it means they are able to communicate an understanding of the patient's experience and needs, with the intention of alleviating suffering or pain (Hojat et al., 2013).

Clinical empathy is necessary for effective patient care (Hojat, Louis, Maio, & Gonnella, 2013) and creating therapeutic caring relationships (Mercer & Reynolds, 2002). Furthermore, Egan (2013) describes empathy as a skill or way of being that are central to forming therapeutic relationships with others.

Mercer and Reynolds (2002) describe three purposes for instilling empathy in therapeutic relationships:

1. Initiating supportive, interpersonal communication in order to understand the perceptions and needs of the patient
2. Empowering the patient to learn, or cope more effectively with his or her environment
3. Reduction or resolution of the patient's problems (p. S9)

Empathy within the Interdisciplinary Team

Supporting teamwork and collaboration within the interdisciplinary team fosters safe, quality care. Caprari et al. (2018) conducted a study on ways to improve teamwork and collaboration through building empathy among the interdisciplinary team. The researchers found improved their experience and collaboration among each other when team members understood each other's needs, goals, and roles. When team members built personal relationships with each other, and understood their actual duties and needs, they felt more confident and trustworthy about their peers.

Active Listening

Active listening is an interactive process between two or more people. In nurse-patient interactions, nurses listen to a message, interpret the meaning, ask questions to clarify the meaning, then share feedback about the message to the patient. Nurses need demonstrate active listening through verbal and non-verbal communication, by asking open-ended questions and actively observing the patient. When the nurse is in a relaxed position, leans slightly forward, maintains eye contact, nods, and restates patient concerns, it shows interest and commitment (Arnold & Boggs, 2019).

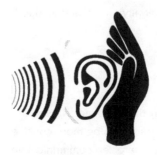

Nurses need to offer their full attention during nurse-patient communication, without making any judgments. Ineffective body language during these interactions can impede message transmission, such as looking at the clock or watch, responding to a text message, or begin walking away from the patient.

Listening makes up 40% of the communication process (Burley-Allen, 2005) and requires the listener to be actively immersed in the dialogue. The listener must be both physically attentive and mentally focused on the spoken message while visibly displaying a relaxed, open-minded body language (Chichirez & Purcărea, 2018).

Van Servellen (2009) explains the following listener responsibilities:

- Perform active listening skills and behaviors
- Understand the message
- Interpret and ask questions about the speaker's body language
- Motivate the speaker to substantiate their message with supports, such as sharing a rationale

Henrico and Visser (2012) expressed the importance of being supportive and genuine during the communication process. An effective listener needs to be concerned about the speaker's feelings and listen in an empathetic way.

Longweni and Kroon (2018) studied the communication process between managers and their employees. The researchers found employees were more engaged and committed when their manager paid attention to their emotions during the communication process. Researchers found employees with lower levels of education perceived less effective communication and required adjustments in communication behaviors. Considering a variety of factors and abilities about the listener will increase the odds of successful communication.

Nurses communicate with interdisciplinary team members and a variety of other staff and employees on a daily basis. Nurses need to listen effectively and be flexible in their communication approach. The goal of effective communication is to empower all involved in the delivery of care.

Consider the following communication skills and behaviors and their impact on effective message transmission:

- **Silence:** opportunity for the patient to interpret the meaning of the message and develop a meaningful response
- **Open-ended questions:** allow for a broader exploration of the patient's situation or concerns
- **Distance reduction:** the amount of physical space varies depending on culture and the nature of the interaction. *More information on physical space in the Communication Barriers section below.*
- **Restating and Clarification:** confirms accurate understanding of the patient's message throughout the dialogue; demonstrates to the patient the nurse is listening and is interested in the dialogue
- **Focusing:** create an environment where the dialogue can be understood clearly, eliminate distractions.
- **Summarizing:** at the end of a dialogue, share a summary of the patient's messages, their needs, concerns, and requests.
- **Collaboration:** encourage patients to be an active participant in their care by communicating needs and concerns, asking questions.
- **Honesty:** honesty and trust coexist. In order to achieve a trusting relationship, honesty and truth telling are required (Bok, 1999). Without honesty, there can be no trust. Additionally, veracity (the ethical principle known as truthfulness) is the foundation for earning another's trust. Pergert and Lutzen (2012) state truth-telling in healthcare is considered a universal communicative virtue. It is important to identify the instances where truth telling is warranted, collaboration with the patient and family at the start of care is necessary.
- **Genuineness:** be yourself, authentic in your daily practice.
- **Respect:** one of the fundamental principles of nursing practice is respect for human dignity, as stated in the ANA (2015a) Code of Ethics, Provision 1: "The nurse practices with compassion and respect for the inherent dignity, worth, and unique attributes of every person" (p. 1).

Communication Tools

Nurses and physicians have different communication styles due to a variety of factors, one being their training. Nurses are educated to share more descriptive accounts of clinical situations compared to physicians who are trained to be more concise in their communication (O'Daniel & Rosenstein, 2008). In order to reduce this communication gap, standardized communication tools have been developed.

Situation-Background-Assessment-Recommendation Tool

In 2002, a group of physicians at Kaiser Permanente developed a communication tool called Situation-Background-Assessment-Recommendation (SBAR) (Sutcliffe, Lewton, & Rosenthal, 2004). The SBAR tool is widely used in healthcare organizations to provide a framework for nurse-physicians communication. The SBAR tool is especially useful in urgent situations when immediate attention and action is critical. The Institute for Healthcare Improvement (IHI, 2020) explains SBAR as follows:

- **S = Situation:** a concise statement of the problem
- **B = Background:** clinical background or context of the problem
- **A = Assessment:** patient data shared, analysis and consideration of options
- **R = Recommendation:** action requested, recommendations shared (para. 1)

O'Daniel and Rosenstein (2008) explains the use of the SBAR tool improves critical thinking for the person (nurse) initiating the communication. When using the SBAR tool, the individual (in this case nurses) needs to assess the problem holistically, then analyze the assessment data, suggest potential underlying causes of the problem, and finally, offer solutions. Using the SBAR tool, or other communication tools, nurses learn how to problem solve in a systematic, holistic way.

Visit the online course to view the video on SBAR.

TeamSTEPPS®

Healthcare facilities have instituted formal approaches using models of care to improve communication, teamwork, and facilitate a more streamlined, and safer delivery of healthcare. The Agency for Healthcare Research and Quality (AHRQ, 2019), in collaboration with the Department of Defense, has created a teamwork system called Team Strategies and Tools to Enhance Performance and Patient Safety (TeamSTEPPS®).

TeamSTEPPS® is an evidence-based approach used to improve communication, safety, and teamwork skills. The TeamSTEPPS® model involves a series of training modules and integration of healthcare principles throughout all areas of the healthcare system (AHRQ, 2019). TeamSTEPPS® improves safety and the quality of care by:

- Producing highly effective medical teams that optimize the use of information, people, and resources.
- Increasing team awareness and clarifying team roles and responsibilities.
- Resolving conflicts and improving information sharing.
- Eliminating barriers to quality and safety (AHRQ, 2019, para. 2)

Clapper et al. (2018) found improved teamwork and communication knowledge as a result of the TeamSTEPPS® training.

Parker, Forsythe, and Kohlmorgen (2019) completed a review of 19 studies assessing the success and influence of TeamSTEPPS® in improving communication, reducing errors, and the impact on patient satisfaction. These studies were focused on outpatient clinic settings and the results of the review found a marked improvement in communication, decrease errors, and improvement in patient satisfaction. Additionally, Clapper et al. (2018) found improved teamwork and communication knowledge as a result of the TeamSTEPPS® training.

Implementing new communication processes requires significant research, planning, administrative support and especially, buy-in from all employees. Shaw et al. (2012) writes about the importance of having a "change champion" on each unit, a critical player who supports innovation and change. Nurses are uniquely positioned to take this role because they are positioned at the center of the interdisciplinary team. Nurses must take the initiative to find gaps in the healthcare delivery process and actively seek out "change" solutions.

Targeted Solutions Tool® for Hand-Off Communication

Hand-off communication has been found to be a contributing factor to adverse events (Scott et al., 2017), wrong-site surgery, delay in treatment, falls, and medication errors (CRICO Strategies, 2015). The Joint Commission for Transforming Healthcare (JCTH, 2020b) has identified inadequate hand-off communication as a sentinel event in healthcare facilities.

The JCTH (2020b) defines hand-off as "a transfer and acceptance of patient care responsibility achieved through effective communication. It is a real- time process of passing patient- specific information from one caregiver to another or from one team of caregivers to another for the purpose of ensuring the continuity and safety of the patient's care" (para. 2). The JCTH (2020) has identified an average of 4000 hand-offs each day in a typical teaching hospital. The opportunity for inadequate communication is vast.

The Joint Commission Resources

Since TJC (2010) required hospitals to implement standardized communication procedures for patient-centered care, they developed a variety of resources, tools, and protocols to assist with improving effective interprofessional communication skills. The following resources assist hospitals with breaking down communication barriers, including cultural, language, and diversity:

- Advancing Effective Communication, Cultural Compentence, and Patient- and Family- Centered Care: A Roadmap for Hospitals
- Hospitals, Language and Culture: A Snapshot of the Nation
- Exploring Cultural and Linguistic Services in the Nation's Hospitals: A Report of Findings
- One Size Does Not Fit All: Meeting the Health Care Needs of Diverse Populations

TJC (2017) also established a hand-off communication procedure as one of the National Patient Safety Goals in 2006, then in 2010 hand-off communication became a Provision of Care standard, as follows:

> The organization's process for hand-off communication provides for the opportunity for discussion between the giver and receiver of patient information. Note: Such information may include the patient's condition, care, treatment, medications, services, and any recent or anticipated changes to any of these (The Joint Commission, 2017, para. 4).

The risk for inadequate discourse and miscommunication is vast, which led the JCTH (2020a) to create the Targeted Solutions Tool® (TST) to improve hand-off communication. The TST provides a framework for improving the effectiveness of communication when a patient moves from one setting to another within the organization or to the community. The TST has the following benefits:

- Increased patient, family, and staff satisfaction
- Successful patient transfers without "bounce back" (patients returning to previous unit)
- Improved safety (JCTH, 2020a)

Benjamin, Hargrave, and Nether (2016) implemented the TST in the Emergency Department to determine the rate of defective handoffs (a TST concept) and the factors that contributed to the handoff. Prior to implementing the TST, the defective handoff rate was 29.9% (32 defective handoffs/107 handoffs). Sixty-nine percent of the contributing factors were uncovered:

- Inaccurate/incomplete information
- Ineffective methods for handoff
- No standardized procedures for handoff
- Lack of patient knowledge of the person initiating the handoff

After implementation of the TST, the defective handoff rate dropped 58% to 12.5% (13 defective handoffs/104 handoffs). As the defective handoff rate declined, the number of adverse events declined.

In a 2015 report, it is estimated that 30 percent of all malpractice claims in U.S. hospitals and medical practices were due to communication failures, resulting in 1,744 deaths and $1.7 billion in malpractice costs over five years (CRICO Strategies, 2015).

Visit the online course to view the video illustrating the breakdown of communication between physicians and patients.

Nurses can bridge this communication gap by identifying and reducing communication barriers within the healthcare team.

Family-Centered Rounds

Khan et al. (2018) implemented a family-centered communication program to reduce errors and improve communication. The outcome of the study reduced harmful medical errors and improved communication processes and family experiences. To view the report and a short video on the study and its outcomes visit the publisher's website.

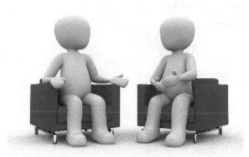

Communication Barriers

Personal Barriers

Holmes, Wieman, and Bonn (2015) conducted a comprehensive review of the research on interprofessional communication and found a number of barriers led to miscommunication, including misunderstood motives, lack of confidence, poor organization, and structural hierarchies. In addition to reduced health outcomes, Storlie (2015) found poor communication impacted not only the patient, but also the healthcare provider and the employer:

Older adults

- chronic elevated levels of stress
- hurt feelings
- delay of care
- dissatisfaction of care

Healthcare provider

- interpersonal conflicts
- health risks
- poor morale
- absenteeism
- burnout
- staff turnover

- reduced quality of care (leading to reduced reimbursement and a poor reputation)
- reduced patient satisfaction (leading to reduced reimbursement and a poor reputation)
- lower staff retention rates leading to increased cost for new hires (Storlie, 2015)

Barriers to communication may originate from the patient or nurse perspective, the physical environment, or the structure of the team dynamics. Nurses can often identify communication barriers among the patient and entire healthcare team and assist individuals on how to reduce miscommunication.

Patient-related barriers

- Preoccupation with pain, discomfort, worry
- Feelings of being judged, insecure, or defensiveness
- Confusion, too much information, complex messages
- Lack of privacy
- Physical barrier: sensory or cognitive deficits

Nurse-related barriers

- Concerned about agenda, heavy workload
- Making assumptions about patient motivations or needs
- Cultural stereotypes
- Insecurity about ability to help patient
- Poor listening/thinking about what to say next (Arnold & Boggs, 2019)

Nurses have an ethical responsibility to prevent personal issues from impacting professional communication (Arnold & Boggs, 2019). Incorporating self-awareness and reflection into practice can assist nurses with reducing communication barriers. Nurses may consider taking a brief "planning pause" before an interaction to remind oneself on the goal of the upcoming communication, to approach the interaction without bias, and consider how non-verbal behaviors may contradict the spoken word.

Interdisciplinary Communication

O'Daniel and Rosenstein (2008) list the following common barriers to interdisciplinary communication and collaboration:

- Personal values and expectations
- Personality differences
- Hierarchy
- Disruptive behavior
- Culture and ethnicity
- Generational differences
- Gender
- Historical interprofessional and intra-professional rivalries
- Differences in language and jargon
- Differences in schedules and professional routines
- Varying levels of preparation, qualifications, and status
- Differences in requirements, regulations, and norms of professional education
- Fears of diluted professional identity
- Differences in accountability, payment, and rewards

- Concerns regarding clinical responsibility
- Complexity of care
- Emphasis on rapid decision-making (para. 12)

Hierarchy

Hierarchy is defined as "the classification of a group of people according to ability or to economic, social, or professional standing" (Merriam-Webster, 2019). This definition applies to different units and professions throughout most healthcare organizations. Hierarchical relationships, such as nurse-physician, novice-to-senior nurse, or other relationships throughout the organization where levels of education, knowledge, or status vary.

Historically, nurses have held subservient roles in their everyday work with physicians. In these situations, physicians are in charge of all decision-making without nursing input leading to poorer quality of care. These hierarchical team structures, where physicians hold a senior position within the team, disempower nurses, resulting in a lack of confidence, fear of humiliation, and the feeling their knowledge and opinions are not valued. Nurses and physicians communicate differently, and while this diversity may offer valuable perspectives and a patient-centered care approach, the fast-paced, complex healthcare environment increases the occurrence of miscommunication (Foronda, MacWilliams, & McArthur, 2016).

Quality patient care is jeopardized when nurses are reluctant to communicate with physicians in order to avoid conflict and fear of repercussions (Gillespie, Chaboyer, Longbottom, and Wallis, 2010). Addressing this dangerous and unsafe communication barrier is crucial to improving communication and reaching optimum patient care outcomes.

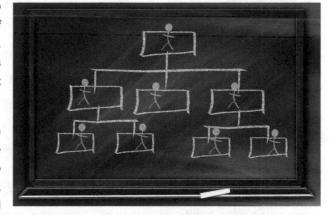

Leadership must approach the negative consequences of a hierarchical team structure with a zero-tolerance policy. To reduce the negative aspects of hierarchy among the team, nurses need to discuss their fears and concerns with management, and together, come up with a plan for remediation. It is the nurse's ethical responsibility to take action, to reduce the impact of hierarchical structures. By collaborating with management, nurses are taking an important step towards improving the delivery of safe, quality patient care.

The following interventions led to improved nurse-physician communication in the ICU setting:

- Daily goal sheet or form
- Bedside whiteboard
- Door communication card
- Team training
- Electronic SBAR documentation templates (Wang, Wan, Lin, Zhou, and Shang, 2017)

Effective listening and receiving unwavering support from management has also been found to reduce the negative impact of hierarchy between nurses and physicians (Lyndon, Zlatnik, & Wachter, 2011)

Interventions can be modified to apply to a variety of healthcare settings. Nurses need to assess gaps in communication at their workplace, take the initiative to find solutions and integrate them into practice. Creating unit or agency policies on the use of communication tools or interventions is a necessary step towards reducing the hierarchical structure of the team, leading to improved nurse-physician collaboration.

Implementation of the TeamSTEPPS® training program has been found to be a powerful tool in reducing hierarchy within an organization. The program provides employees with tools that empower them to voice their concerns, especially in clinical practice situations when patient safety is at risk. When employees are given opportunities to communicate in a safe way, without fear of repercussion or conflict, it minimizes the negative aspects of the hierarchical relationship (Clapper, 2018).

Visit the online course to view the video on nurse-physician communication.

Physical Barriers

Consider the ten major concepts of Nightingale's Environmental theory and how nurses automatically make adjustments to the patient's environment in order to aid in healing, health, improve mood, but also with communicating clearly and accurately with patients:

- Ventilation and warming
- Light and noise
- Cleanliness of the area
- Health of houses
- Bed and bedding
- Personal cleanliness
- Variety
- Offering hope and advice
- Food
- Observation (Pepetrin, 2016)

Assessing the patient's immediate environment is standard nursing practice, though it is important for the nurse to view the environment as a potential barrier to communication. Consider a patient with Chronic Obstructive Pulmonary Disease, with symptoms including shortness of breath, anxiety, restlessness, discouragement, pain, weakness, and activity intolerance. Patients with these symptoms may struggle with a number of environmental factors that could impact sending and receiving messages from others. Patients may struggle with bright or low lights; warm, still air; or a noisy environment.

Lowering the lights, turning on a fan or air conditioning, and reducing the number of visitors can improve comfort, reduce pain or discomfort, ultimately improving the patient's ability to concentrate on nurse-patient interactions and communication more easily.

Papastavrou, Andreou, Efstathiou (2014) found the following environmental barriers negatively impacted communication for stroke patients in an acute care setting:

Provider

- physical characteristics, such as their hearing or speech attitude about caring and respect

Physical environment

- assistive devices (call bell out of reach, lack of hearing aid)
- external sounds
- poor lighting, lack of large print

Hospital procedures

- lack of staff

While this list of barriers was found to be present in a stroke unit, many of them can apply to other units or settings.

Physical Space

DeVito (2016) identifies four ranges of interpersonal space for communication in the United States:

- Intimate relationships: touch to 18 inches
- Personal: 18 inches to 4 feet
- Social: 4-12 feet
- Public: 12-25 feet (p. 152-153)

Arnold and Boggs (2019) state therapeutic communication occurs at 3-4 feet, though more physical space is needed if a patient is anxious. In contrast, less than 3 feet is often used during a painful procedure or injury. Though a patient-centered approach is needed in all situations, assessing for patient preference can prevent miscommunication.

Gender

Men and women differ in many ways in respect to both verbal and non-verbal communication behaviors. Yang et al. (2016) found men tended to stand closer to those of the same gender compared to women. This means women tend to give more space to other women compared to men. Patients and coworkers will find it awkward to tell someone to move back though having the awareness that adequate space is essential for transmission of a message from one person to the other.

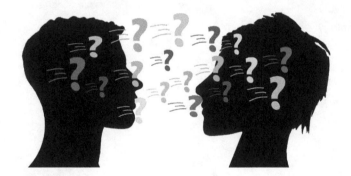

Another gender barrier to communication is verbal communication. How men and women speak can be judged incorrectly. Smith (n.d.) explains the differences in how men and women communicate in Table 1:

Table 1: Gender Differences in Communication

Women	Men
Talk about other people	Talk about tangible things like business, sports, food and drinks
Ask questions to gain an understanding	Talk to give information rather than asking questions
More likely to talk to other women when a problem or conflict arises	Known for dealing with problems or issues internally
Focus on feelings, senses and meaning. They rely on their intuition to find answers	Focus on facts, reason and logic. They find answers by analyzing and figuring things out
Disagreement affects many aspects of their relationship and may take a long time to resolve	Can argue or disagree and then move on quickly from the conflict

Jargon

Subramaniam et al. (2017) defines jargon as the language that is focused on a specific profession or group. Jargon is commonly used during communication by medical professionals, and those who are not familiar with these terms are excluded from the conversation. Examples include "frequent flyer", "trainwreck" and "boyfriend". How would a patient appreciate overhearing a nurse referring to someone as a trainwreck?

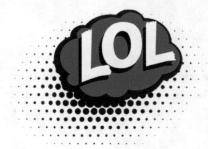

The use of slang is a more casual type of jargon that is not usually used in professional settings, though can occur among nurses and other staff. One popular term is "LOL". As with jargon, those who do not use or know these terms are again excluded from the conversation.

One negative side of slang and jargon is they can have multiple meanings. Consider "LOL", it can mean laugh out loud, lots of love, smiling, amusement, lots of luck, lots of love. While some of these meanings can apply to the same situation, one can see how the intended message can be lost when using a word or phrase with multiple meanings.

The best approach to effective communication is to follow best practices, as follows:

- know your audience
- reduce communication barriers
- monitor non-verbal behaviors and tone of voice
- speak clearly and assertively
- use professional terminology
- listen effectively

Interprofessional Collaboration

Healthcare has faced a vast number of challenges in delivery of quality care over the past 50 years. The population is older, more diverse, medically complex with a higher prevalence of chronic disease requiring multiple specialty providers, a greater reliance on technology and innovation, and uncoordinated delivery systems. Healthcare has also shifted towards delivering care to individuals with vast healthcare disparities (Institute of Medicine [IOM], 2003a). Collaborative practice can improve the delivery of care through a concerted effort from all members of the healthcare team and leaders through the organization.

In response to these challenges, collaborative practice environments are indispensable to improving safety and patient care indicators. Collaborative practice has been found to reduce the rate of complications and errors, reduce length of stay, and lower mortality rates. Collaboration also leads to reduce conflict among staff and reduced turnover. Additionally, collaborative practice strengthens health systems, improves family health, improves infectious disease, assists with humanitarian efforts, and improved response to epidemics and noncommunicable disease (World Health Organization [WHO], 2010).

Collaboration has become an essential component to implementing health promotion and disease prevention/management (Humphreys et al., 2012; Odum & Whaley-Connell, 2012). Due to the high rates of medical errors over the past several decades, interprofessional collaboration has emerged as a pragmatic intervention step that can reduce errors and improve care (Interprofessional Education Collaborative [IPEC], 2016)

Nurses and others healthcare professionals need to work together in order to address challenges that impede progress on improving safety and quality care. The IOM (2015) states, "No single profession, working alone, can meet the complex needs of patients and communities. Nurses should continue to develop skills and competencies in leadership and innovation and collaborate with other professionals in health care delivery and health system redesign" (p. 3).

Common Concept Definitions

- **Elements of Collaboration**

    "Participants from different cultures, high level of interaction, mutual authority, sharing of resources" (Green & Johnson, 2015, p. 5)

- **Interprofessional collaborative practice (IPCP)**

    "When multiple health workers from different professional backgrounds work together with patients, families, and communities to deliver the highest quality of care" (Green & Johnson, 2015; WHO, 2010).

- **Interdisciplinary collaboration (IDC)**

    A team of healthcare practitioners who make a joint, consensus decision about patient care facilitated by regular, face-to-face meetings (Ivey, Brown, Teske, & Silverman, 1988).

    Note: The difference between IPCP and IDC is the former can be applied to multiple categories of "patients" (individual patient and/or family, groups, and communities) whereas the latter is applied exclusively to the patient and/or family.

- **Interprofessional teamwork**

    "The levels of cooperation, coordination and collaboration characterizing the relationships between professions in delivering patient-centered care" (IPEC, 2016, p. 8).

- **Interprofessional team-based care**

  "Care delivered by intentionally created, usually relatively small work groups in health care who are recognized by others as well as by themselves as having a collective identity and shared responsibility for a patient or group of patients (e.g., rapid response team, palliative care team, primary care team, and operating room team)" (IPEC, 2016, p. 8).

- **Interprofessional competencies in health care**

  "Integrated enactment of knowledge, skills, values, and attitudes that define working together across the professions, with other health care workers, and with patients, along with families and communities, as appropriate to improve health outcomes in specific care contexts" (IPEC, 2016, p. 8).

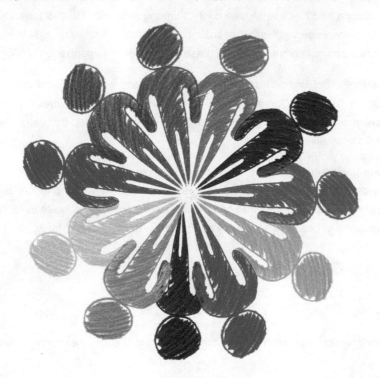

The Institute of Medicine (IOM, 2011) released a landmark report called, *The Future of Nursing: Leading Change, Advancing Health.* The report addressed the critical role of nurses in the delivery of healthcare and made three core recommendations: transforming nursing education, practice, and leadership. The report states nurses must become leaders at every level of the healthcare system in order to participate in ongoing healthcare reform. Leadership is key to becoming a full partner on the healthcare team, and to advocate for policy changes that assist with improving delivery of healthcare.

Additionally, the report found nurses are the best source of information about the patient, family, and communities though are largely excluded from decision-making. Nurses are left with carrying out orders that may or may not be safe, quality patient-centered care. In order to be part of the decision-making process, the report suggests nurses lead through engaging all members of the healthcare team through interprofessional collaboration and mutual respect. The report offers two recommendations in the area of interprofessional collaboration:

Recommendation 2

Expand Opportunities for Nurses to Lead and Diffuse Collaborative Improvement Efforts

Recommendation 7

Prepare and Enable Nurses to Lead Change to Advance Health (IOM, 2011)

The IOM (2015) has followed up on these recommendations and has concluded nursing has made progress with providing quality, patient-centered, accessible, and affordable care, though continued efforts to meet the following recommendations are ongoing:

- Removing barriers to practice and care
- Transforming education
- Collaborating and leading
- Promoting diversity
- Improving data (IOM, 2015)

Benefits of Collaborative Practice

Today's complex healthcare environment has made it difficult for patients to access care, especially those with chronic disease who need access to a variety of specialty services. Patients need assistance with following prescribed orders and follow up appointments with multiple providers. Interprofessional collaboration has improved access to care, safety, chronic disease outcomes, and use of specialty care (Lemieux-Charles & McGuire, 2006; WHO, 2010).

Interprofessional collaboration offers nurses the opportunity to lead and influence change at multiple levels of care (national, regional, local patient settings). Nurses can have a voice in political activism through professional organizations or through academic/practice partnerships (Moss, Seifert, & O'Sullivan, 2016). Collaboration offers nurses the opportunity to serve on boards of directors, government committees, or advisory boards. Through collaboration efforts, nurses can fulfill their role in a variety of ways, with the overarching goal of redesigning the healthcare delivery system.

Through interprofessional collaboration, healthcare organizations can improve safety and quality through committee membership. Nurses can participate in committees that are unit- or organization-wide. Committees are formed based on improving safety and quality by using outcome data, such as preventing hospital-acquired infections, falls, and increased patient satisfaction. Additionally, committees may focus on the health and well-being of staff, to reduce nurse turnover and burnout. Participating in committees benefits everyone, from the patient to the entire organization.

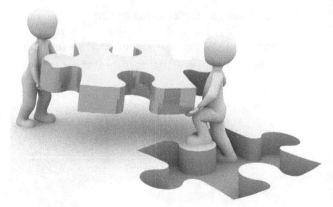

By joining committees, nurses have the opportunity to speak up and share their knowledge and expertise with the interprofessional team, management, and other stakeholders inside and outside of the organization. Interprofessional communication gives nurses a voice, allows them to become intimately involved in the decision-making process and creating solutions. Since nurses implement many of the solutions, nurses must share their insight to ensure the solution has a patient-centered approach. Interprofessional communication is the main way nurses can advocate for and uphold patient rights.

No committees at your workplace? Create one! Locate a problem area in your workplace or unit, research solutions, and present a plan to your manager. Chairing a committee is a good way to network with other professionals and it's an important part of your professional development as a professional nurse

Littlechild and Smith (2013) cite a wide range of healthcare benefits from interprofessional collaboration, including improved efficiency, higher levels of team responsiveness, creative skill sets, and the implementation of innovative holistic services. Several additional benefits of interprofessional collaboration as follows:

- Opportunity to learn new ways of thinking
- Network with professionals from different organizations
- Gain new knowledge, wisdom from others
- Access to additional resources previously unavailable
- Potential to develop new skill sets
- Increased productivity due to shared responsibility
- Access to funding, sharing of costs (research)
- Pooling of knowledge for solving large, complex problems (as cited in Green & Johnson, 2015)

Collaboration has enabled large-scale international organizations like the WHO to achieve more than previously thought possible because of the strength and support of individual members working collectively for a common goal (Green & Johnson, 2015). Collaborations with large groups of professionals and international organizations (such as the WHO) occur throughout all areas of healthcare education, research, and practice. All three domains are connected; research informs education, which informs clinical practice and education. The table below shares some exemplars of successful interprofessional collaboration in healthcare.

Table 1: Exemplars of Successful Interprofessional Collaboration in Healthcare

Name	Purpose	Topic	Website
The Cochrane Collaboration	"Cochrane is a global independent network of health practitioners, researchers, patient advocates and others, responding to the challenge of making the vast amounts of evidence generated through research useful for informing decisions about health."	Evidence	www.cochrane.org
U.S. Preventive Services Task Force	". . . the U.S. Preventive Services Task Force is an independent, volunteer panel of national experts in prevention and evidence-based medicine. The Task Force works to improve the health of all Americans by making evidence-based recommendations about clinical preventive services such as screenings, counseling services, and preventive medications."	Public Health	www.uspreventive servicestaskforce.org
Global Alliance for Musculoskeletal Health	". . . a national and international patient, professional, scientific organisations around the world . . . focused on health policy and evidence, with a mandate to develop strategies and set the agenda, aimed at improving quality of life for individuals around the world by implementing effective prevention and treatment through its unified voice and global reach"	Clinical Practice	https://gmusc.com

Visit the online course to view a TEDx Talks video that discusses the role of collaborative practice in healthcare.

Joy Doll, the speaker in the video mentioned above, discusses six lessons (below) she learned through developing a collaborative practice initiative for a healthcare organization. Joy found these lessons were vital to successful, productive teamwork:

1. Grit: willingness to take on challenges
2. Don't listen to "NO"
3. "Ego-up", engage in meaningful activities that lead towards the goal
4. Psychological safety: speak up with confidence, without consequences
5. Define your culture:
   - everyone teaches, everyone learns
   - assume positive intent of others
6. know yourself through self-assessment, reflection (i.e. strengths/weaknesses)

Joy reflects on the LEGO movie where leadership and collaboration are weaved into the storyline. Find the link to watch the LEGO movie in the online course.

Cost of Reduced Collaboration

The lack of interprofessional collaboration prevents nurses from working to the full extent of their training and education. In order to improve practice, and assist with improving the delivery of healthcare, all nurses must be vested in improving and reducing the barriers of interprofessional collaboration (Moss et al., 2016).

Foundational Documents of Professional Practice

Interprofessional or interdisciplinary collaboration is an indispensable part of nursing practice. The American Nurses Association (ANA, 2015c) defines collaboration as "A professional healthcare partnership grounded in a reciprocal and respectful recognition and acceptance of . . ." (p. 86) the following:

- each partner's unique expertise, power, and sphere of influence and responsibilities
- the commonality of goals
- the mutual safeguarding of the legitimate interest of each party
- the advantages of such a relationship (p. 64)

Scope and Standards of Practice

As discussed in Week 1, the Scope and Standards of Practice, developed by the ANA (2015c), serves as a template for professional nursing practice for all registered nurses. Standard 10, Collaboration, states, "The registered nurse collaborates with the healthcare consumer and other key stakeholders in the conduct of nursing practice" (ANA, 2015c, p. 73). The following is a summary of the competencies of the Collaboration standard:

- Identifies the areas of expertise and contribution of other professionals and key stakeholders.
- Partners with the healthcare consumer and key stakeholders to advocate for and effect change, leading to positive outcomes and quality care.
- Uses effective group dynamics and strategies to enhance team performance.
- Promotes engagement through consensus building and conflict management
- Engages in teamwork and team-building processes (ANA, 2015c, p. 73)

Nursing's Scope of Practice is dynamic and is responsive to the changing needs of individuals and society as a whole. The nursing profession relies on all healthcare professionals to be actively involved in healthcare planning and decision-making, thus collaboration is at the core of all short- and long-term goals (ANA, 2015b). Healthcare professionals are expected to collaborate in the following ways:

- Sharing knowledge, techniques, and ideas about how to deliver and evaluate quality and outcomes in healthcare
- Sharing some functions/duties with others, and having a common focus on the overarching goal
- Recognizing the expertise of others within and outside the profession, referring patients to other providers as appropriate (ANA, 2015b)

The Code of Ethics

As discussed in Week 1, the Code of Ethics is an expression of the values, duties, and commitments of registered nurses. Provision 8 states, "The nurse collaborates with other health professionals and the public to protect human rights, promote health diplomacy, and reduce health disparities" (ANA, 2015a, p. 129). Provision 8 includes two interpretative statements:

8.2: Collaboration for Health Human Rights, and Health Diplomacy

- Nurses are committed to advancing health, welfare, and safety to all people, to individuals and globally. Some examples include world hunger, poverty or environmental pollution, and violation of human rights. Access and availability to quality healthcare services requires interdisciplinary planning and collaboration with partners, whether locally, state-wide, nationally, or globally (ANA, 2015a, p. 203).

8.3: Obligation to Advance Health and Human Rights and Reduce Disparities

- Through collaboration with community organizations, nurses can work individually or collectively, to assist with educating the public on current or future health threats. Nurses have a responsibility to work collaboratively with community agencies to assist the public with facilitating informed choice and identify situations that may contribute to illness, injury or disease. Lastly, the nurse needs to support initiatives that address barriers to healthcare, including the needs of the culturally diverse populations (ANA, 2015a, p. 204)

Provision 2 states, "The nurse's primary commitment is to the patient, whether an individual, family, group, community or population" (ANA, 2015a, p. 25). Interpretive statement 2.3, titled Collaboration, explains shared goal making is a concerted effort of individuals and groups. The complexity of the healthcare system requires nurses to work closely with the interdisciplinary team for safe, quality delivery of care.

Provision of safe, quality care at the community, national, and international levels can be accomplished through creation of community partnerships, political activism and substantial collaboration with all stakeholders. It is the nurse's ethical responsibility to consider collaboration in all aspects of nursing practice. Safe, quality care cannot be performed by one person, but together, with others, goals can be achieved. It is through communication and collaboration that nurses are able to provide the best possible care to their patients.

Nursing's Social Policy Statement

As discussed in Week 1, nursing's social policy statement describes the value of the nursing profession within society, defines the concept of nursing, reviews the standards of practice, and regulation of nursing practice. The nursing practice is inherently connected to society, thus requiring a social contract between society and the profession (ANA, 2015b).

Collaborative efforts with other healthcare professionals are rooted in establishing effective trusting relationships, leading to partnerships where individuals begin to value each other's differences, similarities, experience, and knowledge.

BSN Essentials

Transforming practice to collaborative care environments required transformation of nursing education, as stated in the IOM (2011) report. The BSN Essentials contains nine curricular elements, called Essentials, which provide a framework for baccalaureate nursing education (American Association of Colleges of Nursing [AACN], 2008). Essential VI: Interprofessional Communication and Collaboration for Improving Patient Health Outcomes apples to interprofessional collaboration, as follows:

Communication and collaboration among healthcare professionals are critical to delivering high quality and safe patient care (AACN, 2008, p.3). Collaboration is based on the complementary interaction of the team member's roles. Understanding roles and perspectives are vital to collaboration. The following is a summary of the competencies of a BSN prepared nurse:

- Contribute the nursing perspective to optimize outcomes
- Develop and demonstrate team building and collaborative strategies
- Incorporate effective communication skills to improve team effectiveness
- Consider team member roles, responsibilities, and perspectives during decision-making (AACN, 2008)

Interprofessional Collaborative Practice Organizations

Interprofessional Education Collaborative

The IPEC (2016) was created in 2009 to develop core competencies for interprofessional collaborative practice. The original IPEC report was developed 2011, since revised in 2016, was developed through the initiative of six healthcare disciplines with the intent of defining core interprofessional competencies for their professions. The professions included dentistry, nursing, medicine, osteopathic medicine, pharmacy, and public health. After the release of the first IEC report, support from additional health professions and educational organizations ensued. The four core competencies for interprofessional collaborative practice are as follows:

Competency 1: Values/Ethics for Interprofessional Practice

- Work with individuals of other professions to maintain a climate of mutual respect and shared values.

Competency 2: Roles/Responsibilities

- Use the knowledge of one's own role and those of other professions to appropriately assess and address the health care needs of patients and to promote and advance the health of populations.

Competency 3: Interprofessional Communication

- Communicate with patients, families, communities, and professionals in health and other fields in a responsive and responsible manner that supports a team approach to the promotion and maintenance of health and the prevention and treatment of disease.

Competency 4: Teams and Teamwork

- Apply relationship-building values and the principles of team dynamics to perform effectively in different team roles to plan, deliver, and evaluate patient/population- centered care and population health programs and policies that are safe, timely, efficient, effective, and equitable (IPEC, 2016, p. 10)

While standardized forms of communications improve communication, integrating the constructs of teamwork, collaboration, and the awareness of each team member's roles is crucial to the success of interprofessional communication (IPEC, 2016).

Interprofessional Professionalism Collaborative

The Interprofessional Professionalism Collaborative (IPC, n.d.) was created to develop tools used by healthcare education organizations to assist with developing interprofessional professionalism behaviors within academic curriculum. In addition, researchers us the tools developed by the IPC to advance interprofessional professionalism, a required element of interprofessional collaborative practice. The definition of interprofessional professionalism is as follows:

> Consistent demonstration of core values evidenced by professionals working together, aspiring to and wisely applying principles of, altruism and caring, excellence, ethics, respect, communication, accountability to achieve optimal health and wellness in individuals and communities (Frost et al., 2019; Stern, 2006, p. 15).

The IPC (n.d.) has identified six core interprofessional behaviors:

1. **Communication**
   - Impart or interchange of thoughts, opinions or information by speech, writing, or signs; "the means through which professional behavior is enacted." (Stern 2006)

2. **Respect**

   ○ "Demonstrate regard for another person with esteem, deference and dignity . . . personal commitment to honor other peoples' choices and rights regarding themselves . . . includes a sensitivity and responsiveness to a person's culture, gender, age and disabilities . . . the essence of humanism . . . signals the recognition of the worth of the individual human being and his or her belief and value system." (Stern, 2006)

3. **Altruism and Caring**

   ○ Overt behavior that reflects concern, empathy, and consideration for the needs, values, welfare, and well-being of others and assumes the responsibility of placing the needs of the patients or client ahead of the professional interest (IPC, n.d., para. 4).

4. **Excellence**

   ○ Adherence to, exceeds, or adapts best practices to provide the highest quality care (IPC, n.d., para. 5).

5. **Ethics**

   ○ Consideration of a social, religious, or civil code of behavior in the moral fitness of a decision of course of action, especially those of a particular group, profession, or individual, as these apply to every day delivery of care (IPC, n.d., para.6).

6. **Accountability**

   ○ Accept the responsibility for the diverse roles, obligations, and actions, including self-regulations and other behaviors that positively influence patient and client outcomes, the profession, and the health needs of society (IPC, n.d., para. 7).

Nurses are engaged and motivated to provide the best possible care for their patients. Nurses use their knowledge and expertise to design patient-centered goals. In order to realize these goals, nurses must be leaders throughout the healthcare system, and engage others to participate and be vested in full collaboration with the patient's best interest in mind. Sherman (2015) states the following behaviors helps nurses influence others to foster interprofessional collaboration:

- **Establish your voice:** effective communication and listening skills, address concerns, be perceived as trustworthy
- **Expand networks:** develop relationships with others to form a joint vision
- **Shared accountability:** leads to a sense of community, joint decision-making
- **Empower others:** encourage others to speak up and act

WHO: Interprofessional Education & Collaborative Practice

WHO (2010) has created strategies to improve interprofessional education and collaborative practice to improve health outcomes globally. To make this initiative achievable, WHO has outlined a series of action items policymakers can use to improve their local healthcare systems.

WHO (2010) explains that the overall well-being of a country is centered on maternal and child health. Each day, 1500 women die from complications during pregnancy or childbirth worldwide. Healthcare workers who work together to identify the key strengths of each team member and use those strengths to improve the care of complex health issues, can improve these alarmingly high death rates. Maternal and child health is just one of many complex health problems within society that can be improved through collaborative work environments.

Acute care hospitals conduct morning meetings or interdisciplinary rounds to discuss care practices, plans, discharge. Nurses are uniquely positioned at the center of the interdisciplinary team to monitor information exchange between nursing, medicine, dietary, social work, unlicensed staff, and others. Team collaboration will be most effective when trained team members are fully vested in the organization and are experienced in working as a cohesive team

Developing core competencies is an expectation of all nurses. Seeking out professional development opportunities is an obligation as stated in the Code of Ethics. Provision 5, interpretative statement 5.2 states, the nurse has the responsibility for professional growth and maintenance of competence (ANA, 2010a, p. 159).

Barriers and Promoters to Collaboration

Collaboration among healthcare professionals requires leadership and planning, common goals, and a "teamwork" atmosphere. The literature discussed below reviews an assortment of promoters (actions that enhance collaboration and teamwork) and barriers that impact the success of collaboration. The main take aways include a commitment to work together for a common goal, use of effective communication and collaboration skills, and the initiative to identify and resolve team conflicts.

Choi and Pak (2007) conducted a literature review to determine the promotors, barriers, and approaches to enhance interdisciplinary teamwork. The researchers discovered eight major concepts of teamwork and formulated them within the acronym "TEAMWORK."

See Table 2 for the promoters, barriers, and approaches for each concept are aligned to the acronym, including the "14 C's" for teamwork approaches.

Table 2: Promotors, Barriers, and Approaches for Interdisciplinary Teamwork

	Strategy	Promoting Behaviors	Barriers	The 14 C's of Teamwork
T	Team	• good selection of team members • good team leaders • maturity and flexibility of team members	• poor selection of the disciplines and team members • poor process of team functioning	• Coordination of efforts • Conflict management
E	Enthusiasm	• personal commitment of team members	• lack of proper measures to evaluate success of interdisciplinary work • lack of guidelines for multiple authorship in research publications	• Commitment
A	Accessibility	• physical proximity of team members • Internet and email as a sup- porting platform	• language problems	• Cohesiveness • Collaboration
M	Motivation	• incentives	• insufficient time for the project • insufficient funding for the project	• Contribution
W	Workplace	• institutional support and changes in the workplace	• institutional constraints	• Corporate support
O	Objectives	• a common goal and shared vision	• discipline conflicts	• Confronts problems directly
R	Role	• clarity and rotation of roles	• team conflicts	• Cooperation • Consensus decision-making • Consistency
K	Kinship	• communication among team members • constructive comments among team members	• lack of communication between disciplines • unequal power among disciplines	• Communication • Caring • Chemistry (personality, "good fit")
				(Choi and Pak, 2007)

Management support: need to identify and support change championsSimilar to some of the above points, WHO (2010) has identified the following mechanisms that impact collaborative practice, including:

- Initiative to change the culture of an organization, and oneself
- Individual's attitude towards collaboration

Hierarchical Team Structure

Lancaster, Kolakowsky-Hayner, Kovacich, and Greer-Williams (2015) found a lack of collaboration among physicians, nurses, and unlicensed personnel (UAP) due to hierarchical team structures. While some physicians acknowledged nurses' knowledge and expertise, the study revealed hierarchical, subservient relationships. Nurses and UAPs did not have meaningful discussions about patient needs or care, and physicians viewed themselves as the main decision-maker.

The hierarchical structure of healthcare teams must be addressed in order to improve collaboration and communication among the team members. If unresolved, hierarchy will lead to tension, misunderstandings, and conflicts, burdening the healthcare system with consistent poor outcomes and fragmentation of care.

See more information about hierarchy in the previous chapter on Communication

Nursing leadership has a responsibility to create environments where collaboration can transpire on a daily basis, with full, open participation from all members of the interdisciplinary team. Awareness of the barriers to collaboration, such as unequal power among disciplines (hierarchy), language conflicts, or lack of a "good fit" among team members gives rise to educational opportunities for the organization and/or nursing units. Nurses at all levels of care in the organization are responsible for addressing their personal educational gaps, and encourage the team to seek out competency training.

Awareness of team members' roles assists with having accurate expectations of each other. Since nurses spend the greatest amount of time with patients, they are uniquely positioned to share an abundant amount of important information about the patient, thus, an assertive, effective communication style is warranted during collaborative meetings. Eliminating the hierarchy barriers is key to ensuring nurses have the confidence to speak up without fear of being reprimanded by physicians. advocating for patient needs, ensuring safe, quality care is provided requires an environment where information is shared freely and everyone's voice is heard.

Tools and Frameworks to Improve Interprofessional Collaboration

Morgan, Pullon, and McKinlay (2015) conducted a review of the literature examining the elements of interprofessional collaboration in primary care settings. The overarching element to achieving and sustaining effective interprofessional collaboration was the opportunity to share frequent, informal communication among team members. Continuous sharing of information led to an interprofessional collaborative practice, where knowledge is shared and created among the team members, leading to development of shared goals and joint decision-making. Two key facilitators to interprofessional collaboration are the availability of a joint meeting time to communicate and having adequate physical space.

See the previous chapter on Communication for information on TeamSTEPPS®, an evidence-based tool designed to improve patient safety and quality though improved communication and collaboration.

In Week 4, Leadership in Nursing, discussion about the Healthy Work Environment Model (HWEM), created by the American Association of Critical Care Nurses (AACN, 2016), incorporates *True Collaboration* as one of the six core standards. The *True Collaboration* standard states nurses must be relentless in pursuing collaboration.

See Week 4 for more information about AACNs Healthy Work Environment Model

Successful collaboration is highly valued and a necessity in today's healthcare environment. Experts suggest the daunting process of building a culture of collaboration within an organization is well worth the effort and an indispensable part of success (Adler, Heckscher, & Prusak, 2011).

Critical Thinking

High quality, safe patient care is dependent upon the healthcare provider's ability to reason, think, and make judgments about care. Critical thinking, clinical reasoning and judgment are integral to quality clinical decisions and actions. Today's healthcare landscape has transitioned towards an environment where patients are more medically complex, an aging population with chronic illness, and increased socioeconomic diversity. In order to provide quality patient-centered care, nurses need to develop CT skills in order to provide patients with expert care (Brunt, 2005).

Developing CT is an ethical responsibility of professional nursing practice, and a component for sound clinical judgments and safe decision-making. Thinking in a logical, systematic way, being open to questioning current practice, and reflecting on one's practice regularly are some key features that strengthen nurses' CT skills.

The quality of clinical decision-making is influenced by a number of factors, including experience, level of education, time pressures, and also the culture of the nursing unit (Johansson, Pilhammar, & Willman 2009). Developing critical thinking skills has the potential to improve personal practice and patient outcomes.

Critical thinking (CT) is a process used for problem-solving and decision-making. CT is a broad term that encompasses clinical reasoning and clinical judgment. Clinical reasoning (CR) is a process of analyzing information that is relevant to patient care. When data is analyzed, clinical judgments about care is made. The process of analyzing the data, making decisions is the result of CT—thinking critically throughout the entire patient situation, weighing all relevant options and using CT skills to make the best decision for the patient.

While many definitions have been cited for CT (see below), there is a general agreement that CT is a purposeful action that includes analysis, logical reasoning, intuition, and reflection. Making a concerted effort to critically think during patient care leads to safe, effective decisions. Developing CT skills is key for all nurses, they spend the most time with patients, and are able to recognize subtle changes in their patients and are positioned to make quick, precise decisions, often lifesaving. Using effective CT skills allows nurses to shape the outcome of a patient's experience with the healthcare system.

Critical Thinking definitions

The concept of critical thinking has been an integral part of professional frameworks for generations, yet scholars still debate a universal accepted definition. Dozens of CT definitions have been published, with each of them sharing some common features, such as reflection, contemplation, holism, and intuition. The list below shares a variety of CT definitions:

"The rational examination of ideas, inferences, assumptions, principles, arguments, conclusions, ideas, statement beliefs and action" (Bandman & Bandman, 1995, p. 7)

A reflective skepticism; "reflecting on the assumptions underlying our and others' ideas and actions and contemplative alternative ways of thinking and living" (Brookfield, 1987, p. 18)

"The process of purposeful self-regulatory judgment . . . gives reasoned consideration to evidence, context, conceptualization, methods and criteria: (Facione, 2006, p. 21)

"Reasonable and reflective thinking that is focused upon deciding what to believe or do: (Kennedy, Fisher, & Ennis, 1991, p.46)

"An investigation whose purpose is to explore a situation, phenomenon, question, or problem to arrive at a hypothesis or conclusion about it that integrates all available information and that, therefore, can be convincingly justified" (Kurfiss, 1988, p. 37)

"The propensity and skill to engage in an activity with reflective skepticism" (McPeck, 1961, p. 8)

"The deliberative nonlinear process of collecting, interpreting, analyzing, drawing conclusions about, presenting and evaluating information that is both factual and belief based" (National League for Nursing Accrediting Commission, 2000, p. 8)

"A unique kind of purposeful thinking in which the thinker systematically and habitually imposes criteria and intellectual standards upon the thinking, taking charge of the construction of thinking, guiding the construction of the thinking according to the standard, and assessing the effectiveness of the thinking according to the purpose, the criteria and the standards" (Paul, 1993, p. 21)

"In nursing . . . an essential component of professional accountability and quality nursing care [that exhibits] confidence, contextual perspective, creativity, flexibility, inquisitiveness, intellectual integrity, intuition, open-mindedness, perseverance and reflection." (Scheffer & Ruberfeld, 2000, p. 357)

Concepts Related to Critical Thinking

Clinical Reasoning

- A process where nurses integrate and analyze patient data to make decisions about patient care (Simmons, Lanuza, Fonteyn, & Hicks, 2003)

Clinical Decision-Making

- A process of choosing between different options or alternatives (Thompson & Stapley, 2011)

Clinical Judgment

- A cognitive process used to make judgments based on patient data and cues. Nurses interpret a patient's concerns, needs, and health problems for proper decision-making (Tanner, 2006, p. 204)
- Outcome of critical thinking in nursing practice; judgments begin with the end goal in mind; outcomes are met, involves evidence (Pesut, 2001)

Logical Reasoning

- Arriving at a conclusion based on relatively small amounts of knowledge and/or information (Westcott, 1968)

Intuition

- "Drawing inferences or conclusions that are supported in or justified by evidence (Alfaro-LeFevre, 2015, p. 232)

Reflection

- A purposeful analysis of one's current and past actions (Schon, 1987)

Experience and Clinical Reasoning

According to Benner's (1984) novice to expert model, expert nurses have an intuitive grasp of their patients' problems, their approach is fluid, flexible, and proficient. Compared to novice nurses, they are more task oriented and require frequent verbal and physical cues to provide care.

Novice nurses are challenged with overcoming a knowledge gap, leading to less effective decisions and actions. Compared to experienced nurses, who are challenged with traditional thinking, leading to less effective clinical judgments and decisions (Cappelletti, Engel, & Prentice, 2014). Successful CR and decision-making require a balance of intuition and evidence-based thinking to make effective clinical decisions (Simmons et al., 2003).

Andersson, Klang, and Petersson (2012) found nurses who were specialized in their setting (more experience) used a more holistic approach to making decisions (p. 876), compared to less experienced nurses who used a "task-and action-oriented approach" (p. 873). Gaining experience and knowledge is one way to improve thinking and decision-making, though improving CT skills can close the gap. Being open-minded, self-aware, and reflective offers nurses important information that can improve CR and decision-making. Clinical judgment (akin to CR) improves over time with nurses who uses reflection as a guide for decisions and actions (Cappelletti et al., 2014).

Critical Thinking and Clinical Decision-Making

Lee, Abdullah, Subramanian, Bachmann, and Ong (2017) conducted an integrated review on nine studies to determine whether effective CT impacted clinical decision-making. Four studies found CT impacted decision-making, though five studies did not find a correlation. Due to poor study designs, Lee et al. (2017) could not come to a clear decision on whether there was as significant correlation.

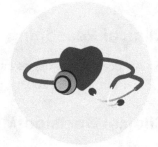

CT continues to be an important factor for problem-solving, regardless if studies can confirm a correlation to decision-making. Developing CT skills, such as reflection, intuition, and logical reasoning, are essential behaviors that lead to a patient-centered approach. Nurses who stop and think about what worked for a patient in the past, may consider the same option again, or may choose an alternative. Considering all possibilities with the patient's best interest in mind is part of CT and making clinical decisions.

Researchers will continue to study the impact of CT on nursing care. Nurse educators will continue emphasize CT in the curriculum and assist students in developing CT skills throughout all levels of education as they offer students tools and methods for problem-solving.

Rubenfeld and Scheffer (2001) explain the essence of CT in nursing practice:

> Critical thinking in nursing is an essential component of professional accountability and quality nursing care. Critical thinkers exhibit these habits of the mind: confidence, contextual perspective, creativity, flexibility, inquisitiveness, intellectual integrity, intuition, open-mindedness, perseverance, and reflection. Critical thinkers in nursing practice the cognitive skills of analyzing, applying standards, discriminating, information seeking, logical reasoning, predicting and transforming knowledge (2001, p. 125).

Standards of Practice

Critical thinking and clinical reasoning are weaved throughout the *Nursing Scope and Standards of Practice* and *Code of Ethics* (American Nurses Association [ANA], 2015c). The nursing process itself, Standards 1-6, are essentially a tool used for clinical reasoning. The standards require core cognitive competencies and guide nurses to use patient data to make effective clinical decisions.

BSN Essentials

Critical thinking and clinical reasoning are integrated throughout the curriculum for baccalaureate nursing education. Essential I: Liberal Education for Baccalaureate Generalist Nursing Practice (American Association of Colleges of Nursing, 2008), states, "Nursing graduates with a liberal education exercise appropriate clinical judgment, understand the reasoning behind policies and standards, and accept responsibility for continued development of self and the discipline of nursing." (p. 11).

Additionally, a liberal arts education exposes nurses to coursework that educates nurses in a variety of general education areas, stating: "Skills of inquiry, analysis, critical thinking, and communication in a variety of modes, including the written and spoken word, prepare baccalaureate graduates to involve others in the common good through use of information technologies, team work, and interprofessional problem solving." (p. 11).

Nurses are taught to approach care holistically, problem-solve in a systematic way by critically examining each element of care. Through careful communication and interprofessional collaboration, critical thinking is expanded as the nurse uses general knowledge, gains experiences, and is open to examining every facet of his or her practice.

Problem-Solving Approaches

Reflective Thinking

Reflection is a powerful tool for recognizing errors in judgment, questioning one's response, and ultimately improving outcomes. Below are two practice examples that illustrate the power of reflective thinking with interprofessional communication and patient care:

Novice and senior nurse communication

- **Problem:** A novice nurse is struggling with inserting IVs just about every shift. One day, the nurse asks the same more experienced nurse for help again. The nurse listens though does not turn around to face the nurse when questioned, and responds in a swift, aggressive way, "I'm swamped, we have no aides today and I'm falling behind with everything. I'll help you when I get time, but it's going to be a while."
- **Impact:** The nurse's patient is at risk for injury without an IV line. The patient may be upset and unsatisfied with care knowing the IV was out for an extended period of time. The nurse feels dejected, does not feel like she is a valued team member, and loses further confidence in her abilities. She considers quitting her job or transferring to another unit.
- **Reflection:** The experienced nurse realizes she was not empathetic to the nurse's needs and impatient and aggressive in her response. She realizes the nurse is new and doesn't have much confidence in her skills yet. She also knows the nurse is probably disappointed in the lack of teamwork and camaraderie. Most of all, she feels bad about disrespecting her coworker.
- **Impact of reflection:** After reflection of the situation, the nurse apologizes for her poor behavior. She states she will work with her each shift they work together, she will share personal tips and review educational materials. Additionally, she will offer to have her observe her IV insertions until she has mastered the skill. She will also make sure the new nurse feels like she is part of the team, not just the new nurse.

Shift report

- **Problem:** The oncoming nurse enters his patient room for the first time and finds the foley bag is full and the patient is complaining of abdominal discomfort.
- **Impact:** The patient is at risk for infection and may be disappointed with the quality of nursing care.
- **Reflection:** The oncoming nurse realizes there is always one or two problems or inconsistencies when he assesses his patients for the first time. He knows the outgoing nurses are skilled and provide quality care and considers another reason

for the errors. After thinking about this for a while, he believes the process for shift report can help reduce change of shift errors. The nurse realizes there needs to be a better way for sharing patient information during change of shift.

- **Impact of reflection:** The nurse researches evidence-based practices to improve safety and quality during shift change. The nurse shares a copy of the review article on bedside report with his manager. The nurse offers to be a change champion on the unit to implement a new process for shift report.

Long-term impact of reflection:

- Improved team cohesiveness, nurse retention and job satisfaction
- Improved patient satisfaction experience and quality of care, leading to higher insurance reimbursement

Glynn (2012) states reflective thinking enhances clinical judgment and gives nurses the opportunity to learn from actual or perceived errors. In regard to the communication scenario, it's through reflection that nurses can think about their behaviors and responses. Reflect on the message for clarity, and whether it was shared in an empathetic and respective way.

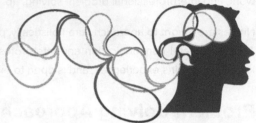

As discussed in the communication chapter, poor communication is the number one reason for medication errors and sentinel events. Through reflection, miscommunication can be identified, solutions found, and implemented. In order for this process to come to fruition, nurses must take the initiative to reflect on their practice.

Creative Thinking

Creative thinking helps nurses generate alternative approaches to clinical decision-making. This type of thinking works especially well with medically complex patients, where care needs to be individualized to reach desired outcomes.

Akin to the concept of "thinking outside the box", finding a novel approach to patient care prevents traditional, stagnant thinking. Choosing alternatives based solely on creative thinking can negatively impact outcomes unless it is paired with the skill of critical thinking. Critical thinking requires the nurse to view the patient holistically,

Intuition

Nurses access knowledge unconsciously and trust this information as fact. Often referred to as a "gut feeling", intuition comes naturally. Intuition is not a tool that is sought out at will, instead the knowledge emerges naturally during a care experience, resulting in firm actions and decisions. Intuition is a measure of professional expertise (Smith, Thurkettle, & Cruz, 2004), a type of clinical judgement that develops over time (Benner, 1984). Since this knowledge is considered intangible or irrelevant, some disregard it, though many studies have shown its positive influence in making accurate decisions and improving the quality of care (Robert, Tilley & Petersen, 2014).

- Nurses will recognize something about their patient that they can't explain, and will make decisions on care without concrete evidence to back up their actions. Such actions can be lifesaving (Billay, Myrick, Luhanga & Yonge 2007). Each clinical experience acts as a learning experience for which lessons are learned and applied to the next experience (McCutcheon & Pincombe, 2001).
- Holtslander (2008) states Carper's (1978) seminal work on the fundamental ways of knowing was published as a reaction to the overemphasis of empirical (scientific) knowledge in nursing practice. One of the four ways of knowing, called *aesthetic knowing,* explains the component of art within nursing practice, an, awareness of the patient, viewing the patient as unique. This viewpoint allows nurses to consider more than just empirical knowledge to guide practice.

Critical Thinking Skills

As discussed earlier, CT encompasses a broad range of reasoning skills that lead to effective decision-making. Through the process of clinical reasoning and judgment, nurses make best choice after assembling and analyzing patient data.

White (2003) studied senior baccalaureate nurses and found the following five themes were essential to developing clinical decision-making skills:

1. Gaining confidence in clinical skills
2. Building relationships with staff
3. Connecting with patients
4. Gaining comfort in self as a nurse
5. Understanding the clinical picture

Scheffer and Rubenfeld (2000) found CT is comprised of affective and cognitive components. Affective components refer to an individual's feelings and attitudes, and cognitive components refer to thought processes. The CT components include 10 habits of the mind (affective components) and seven skills (cognitive components), as follows:

Habits of the mind

- **Confidence:** assurance of one's reasoning abilities
- **Contextual perspective:** considerate of the whole situation, including relationships, background and environment relevant to some happening
- **Creativity:** intellectual inventiveness used to generate, discover, or restructure ideas; imagining alternatives
- **Flexibility:** capacity to adapt, accommodate, modify or change thoughts, ideas, and behaviors
- **Inquisitiveness:** an eagerness to know by seeking knowledge and understanding through observation and thoughtful questioning in order to explore possibilities and alternatives
- **Intellectual integrity:** seeking the truth through sincere, honest processes, even if the results are contrary to one's assumptions and beliefs
- **Intuition:** insightful sense of knowing without conscious use of reason
- **Open-mindedness:** a viewpoint characterized by being receptive to divergent views and sensitive to one's biases
- **Perseverance:** pursuit of a course with determination to overcome obstacles
- **Reflection:** contemplation upon a subject, especially one's assumptions and thinking for the purposes of deeper understanding and self-evaluation (Scheffer & Rubenfeld, 2000, p. 358)

Skills

- **Analyzing:** separating or breaking a whole into parts to discover their nature, function and relationships
- **Applying standards:** judging according to established personal, professional or social rules or criteria
- **Discriminating:** recognizing differences and similarities among things or situations and distinguishing carefully as to category or rank
- **Information seeking:** searching for evidence, facts or knowledge by identifying relevant sources and gathering objective, subjective, historical, and current data from those sources
- **Logical reasoning:** drawing inferences or conclusions that are supported in or justified by evidence
- **Predicting:** envisioning a plan and its consequences
- **Transforming knowledge:** changing or converting the condition, nature, form, or function of concepts among contexts (Scheffer & Rubenfeld, 2000, p. 358)

Development of CT is a lifelong process that requires nurses to be self-aware, and to use knowledge and experience as a tool to become a critical thinker. As nurses move along the continuum from novice to expert, one's competence and ability to critically think will expand (Brunt, 2005).

Evidence-Based Practice

Evidence based practice (EBP) is a problem-solving approach used in the clinical setting. The approach incorporates the use of current evidence from well-designed studies, including the clinician's expertise and patient values and preferences (Melnyk & Fineout-Overholt, 2005). When EBP is used in the context of a caring environment, healthcare providers have improved clinical decision-making and better patient outcomes. Due to the rapid changes in the healthcare system and the complex patient population, healthcare organizations, the federal agencies, and a variety of other organizations, have emphasized the use of EBP in clinical practice (Fineout-Overholt, Melnyk & Schultz, 2005).

The evidence-based practice (EBP) movement began in 1972 when a British epidemiologist, Dr. Archie Cochrane, found the medical profession was not providing care using evidence from systematic reviews (known as strong evidence). Cochrane evaluate current interventions for care and found they were not based on evidence, which led to the creation of The Cochrane Collaboration. The Cochrane Collaboration published systematic reviews that led to the establishment of evidence-based medicine (Shah & Chung, 2009).

As a result of Dr. Cochrane's work, an electronic database was created, known as the Cochrane Library. The primary purpose of the Cochrane organization is to assist healthcare professionals, researchers, and others, in making evidence-based decisions about health care by developing, maintaining, and updating systematic reviews of interventions/treatments and by making these reviews accessible to the public (Cochrane, 2020). For access to systematic reviews, visit the Cochrane Library.

Nurses have been passionate about conducting research since Florence Nightingale's era during the late 1800s. Nightingale's pioneering research during the Crimean War found reduced mortality rates on ill and injured soldiers by improving sanitary conditions and using trained nurses. Nightingale's scientific research findings were presented in her book, *Notes on Nursing*, published in 1860 (McDonald, 2001). Nightingale's work is an example of a nurse having a question about how practice can be altered to improve a clinical problem.

Standards of Professional Practice

Application of EBP is one of the many expectations of professional nursing. As discussed in Week 1, the Scope and Standards of Practice, developed by the American Nurses Association (ANA, 2015c), serves as a template for professional nursing practice for all registered nurses. Standard 13, Evidence-Based Practice and Research, states, "The registered nurse integrates evidence and research findings into practice" (p. 77). The following is a summary of the competencies of the Evidence-Based Practice and Research standard:

- Uses current EBP nursing knowledge, including research findings, to guide practice.
- Incorporates evidence when initiating changes in nursing practice.
- Appraises nursing research for optimal application in practice and the healthcare setting.
- Shares peer-reviewed research findings with colleagues to integrate knowledge into nursing practice (ANA, 2015c, p. 77)

Basic Introduction to Levels of Evidence

The purpose of this basic introduction to levels of evidence is to help the reader differentiate between the different types of research studies. Some research studies are designed to guide practice changes (used as EBP), whereas other studies are used gather new knowledge about a practice topic. The intent of sharing this information is not to gain a thorough understanding of each type of research study, but to have the awareness of which studies are used to guide practice change. You will gain a more thorough understanding of nursing research in NURS 302: Principles of Nursing Research and Evidence Based Practice.

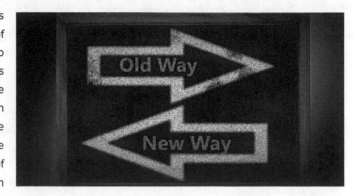

The list below shares seven levels of evidence, ranging from the strongest to the weakest research studies. Studies that share the most reliable information offer *strong evidence* and are referred to as *Level I evidence* (used for EBP). The strength of the research studies are weaker towards the bottom of the list to *Level VII evidence*. The list below shares the definitions for each level of evidence:

Level I: Systematic Review or Meta-Analysis

A synthesis of evidence from all relevant randomized controlled trials.

Level II: Randomized Controlled Trial

An experiment in which subjects are randomized to a treatment group or control group

Level III: Non-Randomized Controlled Trial

An experiment in which subjects are non-randomly assigned to a treatment group or control group.

Level IV: Case-Control or Cohort Study

Case-control study: a comparison of subjects with a condition (case) with those who don't have the condition (control) to determine characteristics that might predict the condition.

Cohort study: an observation of a group(s) (cohort[s]) to determine the development of an outcome(s) such as a disease.

Level V: Systematic Review of Qualitative or Descriptive Studies

A synthesis of evidence from qualitative or descriptive studies to answer a clinical question.

Level VI: Qualitative or Descriptive Study

Qualitative study: gathers data on human behavior to understand *why* and *how* decisions are made.

Descriptive study: provides background information on the *what*, *where*, and *when* of a topic of interest.

Level VII: Expert Opinion or Consensus

Authoritative opinion of expert committee (Fineout-Overholt, Melnyk, Stillwell, & Williamson, 2010).

Developing a basic understanding of the different types of research is the first step to understanding how EPB is generated. For example, using *Level VII evidence* cannot be used to guide practice changes, though it can offer new insights on a topic to stimulate critical thinking and further research.

As discussed earlier integrating research findings is a standard of professional nursing practice. When searching the literature for information on a practice issue, searching the databases for the *strongest* research studies (Level I or II) will offer the nurse valuable information that can be used when considering a practice change.

The scenarios below illustrate which level of evidence is used for a particular need and situation.

Karp, 2019

The nurse manager (NM) of an ICU finds nurses are calling out sick more often, more requests to transfer to different units, and some of the most senior nurses are resigning. The NM wants to learn how to improve retention and create an environment where nurses are satisfied and content in their job and have positive relationships with other nurses and team members. A Level I article offers evidence the NM can use to create a healthy workplace environment. To view an example of a **Level I article, read this article** on job satisfaction among critical care nurses.

A nurse who is new to working at an oncology clinic is interested in understanding the experience of cancer patients undergoing chemotherapy treatment for the first time. To learn more about this topic, the nurse would need to read **Level V or VI** evidence. To view an example of a **Level V or VI article, read this article** to understand cancer patients' experiences.

A staff nurse has been asked to create a presentation on the factors related to opioid-related addiction, drug diversion, and overdose in their unit at the upcoming staff meeting. The nurse can choose an article that offers Level VII evidence if the focus is to share a general overview of the topic. To view an example of a **Level VII article**, an expert panel, **read this article** on on best practices for prescription drug monitoring in the ED setting. If the intent of the presentation is to find evidence to alter practice, a higher level article will be needed, such as Level I or II.

National Institute of Nursing Research

In the mid 1940s, about 80 years after Nightingale published her groundbreaking research, nursing scientists created a formal nursing research program at the federal level, called the Division of Nursing (National Institute of Nursing Research (NINR, n.d.). Federal support for scientific nursing research continued for many years, then in 1985 the research program was renamed to National Institute of Nursing Research (NINR, n.d.), and is now a division of the National Institutes of Health (NIH). The NINR conducts high level scientific research on a wide variety of healthcare issues, offers research funding opportunities, grant and research training, and more. The following is a brief list of the extraordinary research conducted by nurse researchers at NINR:

- Palliative Care Intervention Improves Well-being of Cancer Patients and their Caregivers in Community Practice Setting
- Identification of a Potential Blood-based Biomarker for Diagnosing Mild Traumatic Brain Injuries
- Brain Imaging Shows that Damage Caused by Sleep Apnea Differs by Sex
- Micronutrient Deficiencies are Associated with Poor Heart Failure Outcomes

- Microbiome Associated with Differences in Symptoms and Quality of Life in Women with Irritable Bowel Syndrome

Nurses can ask the following questions and search for research evidence to find answers:

- What can I do to prevent falls for peri-natal patients?
- What is most important to patients when they are admitted to the hospital?
    - Hot food?
    - Pain control?
    - Fast response to a call light?
- Is it okay to test the foley catheter balloon prior to insertion?
- Why do nurses fear repercussions from doctors during communication?
- What can a new nurse do to successfully transition to nursing practice without being bullied by their peers?
- Is a BSN education worth the time and money?
- Are ADN grads equally as competent as BSN grads?
- Why do I have to perform regular mouth care for ventilated patients?
- When is hand sanitizer just as good as soap and water?
- Does specialty certification improve patient outcomes?

These and other common questions can be answered using research evidence. By using the correct level of evidence, nurses can inform practice by improving outcomes, quality, and patient satisfaction, improve nurse morale and reduce burnout, or simply obtain a better understanding of a variety of topics relevant to nursing practice. Taking control of one's practice, and instituting change based on research evidence is crucial to performing at one's highest potential. Seeking out opportunities to learn and share knowledge with peers is essential for the nursing profession.

Barriers and Facilitators to Implementation of EBP

There are a multitude of barriers for implementing EBP, from lack of knowledge, motivation, access to databases, poor technology, lack of time and interest, and the list goes on. Some barriers can be modified though training and mentoring, others require a more focused approach during nursing education training. In order for EBP to take hold within the nursing profession, a concerted effort to from the nurse and the organization is needed.

Solomons and Spross (2011) conducted a review of the literature to determine the barriers and facilitators of implementing of EBP. The following shares an exhaustive list of barriers from the nurse, manager, and organization level:

Barriers

Nurse:

- time constraints
- lack of resources
- demanding workload, high acuity of patients
- performing EBP takes too long
- resistant to change
- lack of authority to change practice
- lack of respect for research
- "doesn't apply to what I do", "not related to bedside care" and "nurses are not trained to think deductively"
- lack of training to participate effectively in multidisciplinary teams
- difficulty accessing resource materials
- lack of confidence in evaluating the quality of the research

- lack of information-seeking skills
- lack of understanding of online research databases such as CINAHL and MEDLINE
- Using Google or Yahoo! for a literature search rather than the scientific research databases
- Difficulty understanding the analysis, statistics found in the research studies
- found research to be overwhelming
- Lack of awareness of research
- too many journals (Solomons & Spross, 2011, pp. 115-117)

Management:

- EBP is not a priority
- lack of infra-structure for research-related activities
- resistant to change
- perceived that nurses were not interested or ready to adopt EBP
- would not be possible to adopt EBP, lack of authority to change practice (Solomons & Spross, 2011, pp. 115-117)

Organization:

- information systems are not powerful enough to support EBP efforts
- poor information systems
- hospital blocked access to online bibliographic databases and other online resources
- lack of a library (Solomons & Spross, 2011, pp. 115-117)

Facilitators

- integrate EBP philosophy and skills into job descriptions and clinical ladders for promotion
- have a nursing presence on hospital-wide committees that support EBP
- incorporate EBP into new employee orientation
- give nurses time during the workday to read and develop practice change activities
- management includes the definition of EBP in all communications
- offer resources for EBP training
- create an EBP council or committee, members should assume leadership roles
- create a newsletter for the organization to disseminate research activities and the importance of EBP
- develop EBP champions throughout the organization, aimed at cultivating staff interest and ownership in research
- attend an annual research symposium
- reward staff for critical thinking
- develop a culture of respect across all disciplines
- hands-on training sessions on how to access and interpret research, develop a manual for nurses
- for a subcommittee to promote the use of EBP among nurses
- include time devoted to learning and understanding research into monthly meetings
- quarterly research workshops and yearly grand rounds
- convert research findings into a format that is easy to understand
- share research knowledge through email and online forums
- use a bulletin board to display current EBP (Solomons & Spross, 2011, pp. 115-117)

References

Adler, P., Heckscher, C., & Prusak., L. (2011, July-August). *Building collaborative enterprise. Harvard Business Review, 89*(7–8), 1-9. https://hbr.org/2011/07/building-a-collaborative-enterprise

Agency for Healthcare Research and Quality. (2019). *About TeamSTEPPS*. http://www.ahrq.gov/teamstepps/about-teamstepps/index.html

Alfaro-LeFevre, R. (2015). *Critical thinking, clinical reasoning, and clinical judgment. A practical approach*. Elsevier Health Sciences.

American Association of Colleges of Nursing. (2008). *The essentials of baccalaureate education for professional nursing practice*. https://www.aacnnursing.org/Portals/42/Publications/BaccEssentials08.pdf

American Association of Critical-Care Nurses. (2016). *AACN standards for establishing and sustaining healthy work environments. A journey to excellence*. (2nd ed.). Author.

American Nurses Association. (2015a). *Guide to the code of ethics for nurses with interpretive statements* (2nd ed.). Author.

American Nurses Association. (2015b). *Guide to nursing's social policy statement. Understanding the profession from social contract to social covenant*. Author.

American Nurses Association. (2015c). *Scope and standards of practice* (3rd ed.). Author.

Andersson, N., Klang, B., & Petersson, G. (2012). Differences in clinical reasoning among nurses working in highly specialized paediatric care. *Journal of Clinical Nursing, 21*(5-6), 870-879. http://doi.org/10.1111/j.1365-2702.2011.03935.x

Arnold, E. C., & Boggs, K. U. (2019). *Professional communication skills for nurses* (8th ed.). Elsevier.

Bandman, E. L., & Bandman, B. (1995). *Critical thinking in nursing* (2nd ed.). Appleton & Lange.

Battié, E. R., & Steelman, V. M. (2014). Accountability in nursing practice: Why it is important for patient safety. *AORN Journal, 100*(5), 537-541. http://doi.org/doi:10.1016lj.aorn.2014.08.008

Benbenishty, J. S., & Hannink, J. R. (2015). Non-verbal communication to restore patient–provider trust. *Intensive Care Medicine, 41*(7), 1359-1360. http://doi.org/10.1007/s00134-015-3710-8

Benjamin, M. F., Hargrave, S., & Nether, K. (2016). Using the Targeted Solutions Tool to improve emergency department handoffs in a community hospital. *The Joint Commission Journal on Quality and Patient Safety, 42*(3), 107-118. http://doi.org/10.1016/S1553-7250(16)42013-1

Benner, P. (1984). *From novice to expert: Power and excellence in nursing practice*. Addison-Wesley.

Billay, D., Myrick, F., Luhanga, F., & Yonge, O. (2007). A pragmatic view of intuitive knowledge in nursing practice. *Nursing Forum, 42*(3), 147-155. http://doi.org/10.1111/j.1744-6198.2007.00079.x

Bok, S. (1999). *Lying: Moral choice in public and private life*. Vintage Books.

Brookfield, S. D. (1995). *Becoming a critically reflective teacher*. Jossey-Bass.

Brunt, B. A. (2005). Critical thinking in nursing: An integrated review. *The Journal of Continuing Education in Nursing, 36*(2), 60-67. http://doi.org/10.3928/0022-0124-20050301-05

Burley-Allen, M. (2005). *Listening: The forgotten skill* (2nd ed.). Wiley.

Cappelletti, A., Engel, J. K., & Prentice, D. (2014). Systematic review of clinical judgment and reasoning in nursing. *Journal of Nursing Education, 53*(8), 453-458. http://doi.org/10.3928/01484834-20140724-01

Caprari, E., Porsius, J. T., D'Olivo, P., Bloem, R. M., Vehmeijer, S. B. W., Stolk, N., & Melles, M. (2018). Dynamics of an orthopaedic team: Insights to improve teamwork through a design thinking approach. *Work, 61*(1), 21–39. http://doi.org/10.3233/WOR-182777

Carper, B.A. (1978). Fundamental patterns of knowing in nursing. *Advances in Nursing Science, 1*(1), 13-24.

Chichirez, C. M., & Purcărea, V. L. (2018). Interpersonal communication in healthcare. *Journal of Medicine and Life, 11*(2), 119-122.

Choi, B. C., & Pak, A. W. (2007). Multidisciplinarity, interdisciplinarity, and transdisciplinarity in health research, services, education and policy: 2. Promotors, barriers, and strategies of enhancement. *Clinical & Investigative Medicine, 30*(6), 224-232. http://doi.org/10.25011/cim.v30i6.2950

Clapper, T. C., Ching, K., Mauer, E., Gerber, L. M., Lee, J. G., Sobin, B.,Ciraolo, K., Osorio, S. N., & DiPace, J. I. (2018). A saturated approach to the four-phase, brain-based simulation framework for TeamSTEPPS® in a pediatric medicine unit. *Pediatric Quality & Safety, 3*(4), 1-7. http://doi.org/10.1097/pq9.0000000000000086

Clapper, T. C. (2018). TeamSTEPPS® is an effective tool to level the hierarchy in healthcare communication by empowering all stakeholders. *Journal of Communication in Healthcare, 11*(4), 241–244. http://doi.org/10.1080/17538068.2018.1561806

Cochrane. (2020). *About us.* https://www.cochrane.org/about-us

Colthorpe, K., Sharifirad, T., Ainscough, L., Anderson, S., & Zimbardi, K. (2018). Prompting undergraduate students' metacognition of learning: Implementing 'meta-learning 'assessment tasks in the biomedical sciences. *Assessment & Evaluation in Higher Education, 43*(2), 272-285. https://doi.org/10.1080/02602938.2017.1334872

CRICO Strategies. (2015). *Malpractice risks in communication failures.* https://www.rmf.harvard.edu/Malpractice-Data/Annual-Benchmark-Reports/Risks-in-Communication-Failures

DeVito, J. A. (2016). *The interpersonal communication book* (14th ed.). Pearson.

Egan, G. (2013). *The skilled helper: A problem-management and opportunity-development approach to helping.* Cengage Learning.

ElaN Holding. (2012, May 8). *Cultural differences in body language.* [video]. YouTube. https://www.youtube.com/watch?v=W3CN3fd2G_E

Facione, P. A. (2006). *Critical thinking: What it is and why it counts.* California Academic Press.

Fineout-Overholt, E., Melnyk, B. M., & Schultz, A. (2005). Transforming health care from the inside out: Advancing evidence-based practice in the 21st century. *Journal of Professional Nursing, 21*(6), 335–344. http://doi.org/10.1016/j.profnurs.2005.10.005

Fineout-Overholt, E., Melnyk, B. M., Stillwell, S. B., & Williamson, K. M. (2010). Evidence-based practice step by step: critical appraisal of the evidence: Part I. *The American Journal of Nursing, 110*(7), 47-52. http://doi.org/10.1097/01.NAJ.0000383935.22721.9c

Foronda, C., MacWilliams, B., & McArthur, E. (2016). Interprofessional communication in healthcare: An integrative review. *Nurse Education in Practice, 19*, 36–40. http://doi.org/10.1016/j.nepr.2016.04.005

Foundation for Critical Thinking. (2019). *Our mission*. http://www.criticalthinking.org/pages/our-mission/405

Frost, J. S., Hammer, D. P., Nunez, L. M., Adams, J. L., Chesluk, B., Grus, C., Harvison, N., McGuinn, K., Mortensen, L., Nishimoto, J. H., Palatta, A. Richmond, M., Ross, E. J., Tegzes, J., Ruffin, A. L., & Bentley, J. P. (2019). The intersection of professionalism and interprofessional care: Development and initial testing of the interprofessional professionalism assessment (IPA). *Journal of Interprofessional Care, 33*(1), 102-115. http://doi.org/10.1080/13561820.2018.1515733

Gillespie, B. M., Chaboyer, W., Longbottom, P., & Wallis, M. (2010). The impact of organisational and individual factors on team communication in surgery: a qualitative study. *International journal of nursing studies, 47*(6), 732-741. http://doi.org/10.1016/j.ijnurstu.2009.11.001

Glynn, D.M. (2012). Clinical judgment development using structured classroom reflective practice: A qualitative study. *Journal of Nursing Education, 51,* 134-139. http://doi.org/10.3928/01484834-20120127-06

Green, B. N., & Johnson, C. D. (2015). Interprofessional collaboration in research, education, and clinical practice: Working together for a better future. *Journal of Chiropractic Education, 29*(1), 1-10. http://doi.org/10.7899/JCE-14-36

Henrico, A., & Visser, K. (2012). Leading. In S. Botha & S. Musengi (Eds.), *Introduction to business management – Fresh perspective* (pp. 160–189). Pearson

Hojat, M., Louis, D. Z., Maio, V., & Gonnella, J. S. (2013). Empathy and health care quality. *American Journal of Medical Quality, 28*(1), 6–7. http://doi.org/10.1177/1062860612464731

Holmes, N. G., Wieman, C. E., & Bonn, D. A. (2015). Teaching critical thinking. *Proceedings of the National Academy of Sciences, 112*(36), 11199-11204. http://doi.org/10.1073/pnas.1505329112

Holtslander, L. (2008). Ways of knowing: Carper's fundamental patterns as a guide for hope research with bereaved palliative caregivers. *Nursing Outlook, 56*(2), 25-30. http://doi.org/10.1016/j.outlook.2007.08.001

Hosley, J., & Molle, E. (2006). *A practical guide to therapeutic communication for health professionals*. Saunders Elsevier.

Humphreys, J., Harvey, G., Coleiro, M., Butler, B., Barclay, A., Gwozdziewicz, M., O'Donoghue, D., & Hegarty, J. (2012). A collaborative project to improve identification and management of patients with chronic kidney disease in a primary care setting in Greater Manchester. *BMJ Quality & Safety, 21*(8), 700-708. http://doi.org/10.1136/bmjqs-2011-000664

Institute for Healthcare Improvement. (2020). *SBAR tool: Situation-Background-Assessment-Recommendation*. http://www.ihi.org/resources/Pages/Tools/SBARToolkit.aspx

Institute of Medicine. (2003a). *The future of the public's health in the 21st Century*. National Academies Press.

Institute of Medicine (2003b). *Health professions education: A bridge to quality*. National Academies Press.

Institute of Medicine. (2011). *The future of nursing: Leading change advancing health*. National Academies Press.

Institute of Medicine. (2015). *Assessing progress on the Institute of Medicine Report The Future of Nursing*. National Academies Press.

Interprofessional Education Collaborative. (2016). *Core competencies for interprofessional collaborative practice: 2016 update*. Author.

Ivey, S. L., Brown, K. S., Teske, Y., & Silverman, D. (1988). A model for teaching about interdisciplinary practice in health care settings. *Journal of Allied Health, 17*(3), 189-195. https://pubmed.ncbi.nlm.nih.gov/3192484/

Johansson, M.E., Pilhammar, E., & Willman, A. (2009). Nurses' clinical reasoning concerning management of peripheral venous cannulae. *Journal of Clinical Nursing, 18,* 3366-3375. http://doi.org/10.1111/j.1365-2702.2009.02973.x

Joint Commission for Transforming Healthcare. (2020a). *Hand-off communications targeted solutions tool.* https://www.centerfortransforminghealthcare.org/what-we-offer/targeted-solutions-tool/hand-off-communications-tst

Joint Commission for Transforming Healthcare. (2020b). *Take 5: Tackling inadequate hand-off communication.* https://www.centerfortransforminghealthcare.org/why-work-with-us/podcasts/take-5-tackling-inadequate-hand-off-communication

Joint Commission on Accreditation of Healthcare Organizations. (2005). *The Joint Commission guide to improving staff communication.* Joint Commission Resources.

Joint Commission on Accreditation of Healthcare Organizations. (2009). *The Joint Commission guide to improving staff communication* (2nd ed.). Joint Commission Resources.

Kennedy, M., Fisher, M. B., & Ennis, R. H. (1991). Critical thinking: Literature review and needed research. In L. Idol & B. F. Jones (Eds.), *Educational values and cognitive instruction: Implications for reform and cognitive instruction: Implications for reform* (pp. 11-40). Lawrence Erlbaum.

Khan, A., Spector, N. D., Baird, J. D., Ashland, M., Starmer, A. J., Rosenbluth, G., Garcia, B. M., Litterer, K. P., Rogers, J. E., Dalal, A. K., Lipsitz, S., Yoon, C. S, Zigmont, K. R., Guiot, A., O'toole, J. K., Patel, A., Bismilla, Z., Coffey, M., Langrish, K., . . . Blankenburg, R. L. (2018). Patient safety after implementation of a coproduced family centered communication programme: Multicenter before and after intervention study. *British Medical Journal, 363*(8179), 4995. http://doi.org/10.1136/bmj.k4764

Kurfiss, J. (1988). *Critical thinking, theory, research and possibilities.* Association for the Study of Higher Education.

Lancaster, G., Kolakowsky-Hayner, S., Kovacich, J., & Greer-Williams, N. (2015). Interdisciplinary communication and collaboration among physicians, nurses, and unlicensed assistive personnel. *Journal of Nursing Scholarship, 47*(3), 275-284. http://doi.org/10.1111/jnu.12130

Lee, D. S., Abdullah, K. L., Subramanian, P., Bachmann, R. T., & Ong, S. L. (2017). An integrated review of the correlation between critical thinking ability and clinical decision-making in nursing. *Journal of Clinical Nursing, 26*(23-24), 4065-4079. http://doi.org/10.1111/jocn.13901

Leininger, M. & McFarland, M. (2006). *Cultural care diversity and universality: A worldwide theory for nursing* (2nd ed.). Jones & Bartlett.

Lemieux-Charles, L., & McGuire, W. L. (2006). What do we know about health care team effectiveness? A review of the literature. *Medical Care Research and Review, 63*(3), 263-300. http://doi.org/10.1177/1077558706287003

Littlechild, B., & Smith, R. (2013). *A handbook for interprofessional practice in the human services: Learning to work together.* Routledge.

Longweni, M., & Kroon, J. (2018). Managers' listening skills, feedback skills and ability to deal with interference: A subordinate perspective. *Acta Commercii, 18*(1), 1-12. http://doi.org/10.4102/ac.v18i1.533

Lyndon, A., Zlatnik, M. G., & Wachter, R. M. (2011). Effective physician-nurse communication: A patient safety essential for labor and delivery. *American Journal of Obstetrics and Gynecology, 205*(2), 91-96. http://doi.org/10.1016/j.ajog.2011.04.021

McCutcheon, H. H., & Pincombe, J. (2001). Intuition: An important tool in the practice of nursing. *Journal of Advanced Nursing, 35*(3), 342-348. http://doi.org/10.1046/j.1365-2648.2001.01882.x

McPeck, J. E. (1981). *Critical thinking and education.* St. Martin's Press.

Melnyk, B. M., & Fineout-Overholt, E. (2005). Making a case for evidence-based practice. In B. M. Melnyk, & E. Fineout-Overholt (Eds.), *Evidence-based practice in nursing and healthcare: A guide to best practice* (pp. 3 – 24). Lippincott, Williams & Wilkins.

Merriam-Webster. (2019). *Hierarchy.* https://www.merriam-webster.com/dictionary/hierarchy

Melnyk, B. M., & Fineout-Overholt, E. (2015). *Evidence-based practice in nursing & healthcare* (3rd ed.). Lippincott, Williams, & Wilkins.

Mercer, S. W. & Reynolds, W. J. (2002). Empathy and quality of care. *British Journal of General Practice,* 52(Supplement 1), 9-12.

Morgan, S., Pullon, S., & McKinlay, E. (2015). Observation of interprofessional collaborative practice in primary care teams: An integrative literature review. *International Journal of Nursing Studies, 52*(7), 1217–1230. http://doi.org/10.1016/j.ijnurstu.2015.03.008

Moss, E., Seifert, P. C., & O'Sullivan, A. (2016). Registered nurses as interprofessional collaborative partners: Creating value-based outcomes. *The Online Journal of Issues in Nursing, 21*(3). http://doi.org/10.3912/OJIN.Vol21No03Man04

National Institute of Nursing Research. (n.d.). *History.* https://www.ninr.nih.gov/aboutninr/history

National League for Nursing Accrediting Commission. (2000). *Guidelines for nursing program accreditation.* Author.

O'Daniel, M., & Rosenstein. (2008). Professional communication and team collaboration. In R. G. Hughes (Eds.), *Patient safety and quality: An evidence-based handbook for nurses.* https://www.ncbi.nlm.nih.gov/books/NBK2637/

Odum, L., & Whaley-Connell, A. (2012). The role of team-based care involving pharmacists to improve cardiovascular and renal outcomes. *Cardiorenal Medicine, 2*(4), 243-250. http://doi.org/10.1159/000341725

Omura, M., Maguire, J., Levett-Jones, T., & Stone, T. E. (2016). Effectiveness of assertive communication training programs for health professionals and students: A systematic review protocol. *JBI Database of Systematic Reviews and Implementation Reports, 14*(10), 64-71. http://doi.org/10.11124/JBISRIR-2016-003158

Oyetunde, M. O., & Brown, V. B. (2012). Professional accountability: Implications for primary healthcare nursing practice. *JONA's Healthcare Law, Ethics & Regulation, 14*(4), 109-114. http://doi.org/10.1097/JHL.0b013e318276308f

Papastavrou, E., Andreou, P., & Efstathiou, G. (2014). Rationing of nursing care and nurse–patient outcomes: A systematic review of quantitative studies. *The International Journal of Health Planning and Management, 29*(1), 3-25. http://doi.org/10.1002/hpm.2160

Parker, A. L., Forsythe, L. L., & Kohlmorgen, I. K. (2019). TeamSTEPPS®: An evidence-based approach to reduce clinical errors threatening safety in outpatient settings: An integrative review. *Journal of Healthcare Risk Management, 38*(4), 19–31. http://doi.org/10.1002/jhrm.21352

Paul, R. (1993), *Critical thinking: What every person needs to survive in a rapidly changing world* (3rd ed.). Foundation for Critical Thinking.

Pergert, P., & Lutzen, K. (2012). Balancing truth-telling in the preservation of hope: A relational ethics approach. *Nursing Ethics,* (1), 21-29. https://doi.org/10.1177/0969733011418551

Pepetrin, A. (2016). *Environmental theory.* http://www.nursing-theory.org/theories-and-models/nightingale-environment-theory.php

Peplau, H. E. (1960). Talking with patients. *The American Journal of Nursing, 60*(7), 964-966. http://doi.org/10.2307/3418512

Pesut, J. (2001). Clinical judgment: Foreground/background. *Journal of Professional Nursing, 17*(5), 215. http://doi.org/10.1053/jpnu.2001.26303

Plonien, C. (2015). Using personality indicators to enhance nurse leader communication. *AORN Journal, 102*(1), 74–80. http://doi.org/10.1016/j.aorn.2015.05.001

Ramezani-Badr, F., Nasrabadi, A.N., Yekta, Z.P., & Taleghani, F. (2009). Strategies and criteria for clinical decision making in critical care nurses: A qualitative study. *Journal of Nursing Scholarship, 41,* 351-358. http://doi.org/10.1111/j.1547-5069.2009.01303.x

Robert, R. R., Tilley, D. S., & Petersen, S. (2014). A power in clinical nursing practice: concept analysis on nursing intuition. *Medsurg Nursing, 23*(5). https://pubmed.ncbi.nlm.nih.gov/26292448/

Rosenberg, S., & Gallo-Silver, L. (2011). Therapeutic communication skills and student nurses in the clinical setting. *Teaching and Learning in Nursing, 6*(1), 2-8. http://doi.org/10.1016/j.teln.2010.05.003

Scheffer, B. K., & Rubenfeld, M. G. (2000). A consensus statement on critical thinking in nursing. *Journal of Nursing Education, 39*(8), 352-359. http://doi.org/10.3928/0148-4834-20001101-06

Schon, D. A. (1987). *The reflective practitioner.* Temple Smith.

Scott, A. M., Li, J., Oyewole-Eletu, S., Nguyen, H. Q., Gass, B., Hirschman, K. B., ... & Project ACHIEVE Team. (2017). Understanding facilitators and barriers to care transitions: Insights from Project ACHIEVE site visits. *The Joint Commission Journal on Quality and Patient Safety, 43*(9), 433-447. doi: 10.1016/j.jcjq.2017.02.012

Shah, H. M., & Chung, K. C. (2009). Archie Cochrane and his vision for evidence-based medicine. *Plastic and Reconstructive Surgery, 124*(3), 982-988. http://doi.org/10.1097/PRS.0b013e3181b03928

Shaw, E. K., Howard, J., West, D. R., Crabtree, B. F., Nease, D. E., Tutt, B., & Nutting, P. A. (2012). The role of the champion in primary care change efforts: From the State Networks of Colorado Ambulatory Practices and Partners (SNOCAP). *Journal of the American Board of Family Medicine, 25*(5), 676. http://doi.org/10.3122/jabfm.2012.05.110281

Sherman, R. O. (2015, December 8). Boosting your influence. *American Nurse Today, 10*(12). https://www.myamericannurse.com/boosting-influence/

Simmons, B., Lanuza, D., Fonteyn, M., & Hicks, F. (2003). Clinical reasoning in experienced nurses. *Western Journal of Nursing Research, 25*(6), 701–719. http://doi.org/10.1177/0193945903253092

Smith, C. (n.d.). *The seven barriers of communication. https://guides.co/g/the-seven-barriers-of-communication/37295*

Smith, A. J., Thurkettle, M. A., & Cruz, F. A. D. (2004). Use of intuition by nursing students: Instrument development and testing. *Journal of advanced Nursing, 47*(6), 614-622. http://doi.org/10.1111/j.1365-2648.2004.03149.x

Solomons, N. M., & Spross, J. A. (2011). Evidence-based practice barriers and facilitators from a continuous quality improvement perspective: An integrative review. *Journal of Nursing Management, 19*(1), 109-120. http://doi.org/10.1111/j.1365-2834.2010.01144.x

Stern, D. T. (2006). *Measuring medical professionalism.* Oxford University Press.

Storlie, T. A. (2015). *Person-centered communication with older adults: The professional provider's guide.* Elsevier.

Street Jr, R. L., & Mazor, K. M. (2017). Clinician–patient communication measures: Drilling down into assumptions, approaches, and analyses. *Patient education and counseling, 100*(8), 1612-1618. http://doi.org/10.1016/j.pec.2017.03.021

Subramaniam, R., Sanjeev, R., Kuruvilla, S., Joy, M. T., Muralikrishnan, B., & Paul, J. (2017). Jargon: A barrier in case history taking? A cross-sectional survey among dental students and staff. *Dental Research Journal, 14*(3), 203. https://www.ncbi.nlm.nih.gov/pmc/articles/PMC5504873/

Sutcliffe, K. M., Lewton, E., & Rosenthal, M. M. (2004). Communication failures: an insidious contributor to medical mishaps. *Academic Medicine, 79*(2), 186-194. http://doi.org/10.1097/00001888-200402000-00019

Tanner, C. A. (2006). Thinking like a nurse: A research-based model of clinical judgment in nursing. *Journal of Nursing Education, 45*(6). http://doi.org/10.3928/01484834-20060601-04

TED-Ed. (2016, February 16). *How miscommunication happens (and how to avoid it) – Katherine Hampsten.* [video]. YouTube. https://www.youtube.com/watch?v=gCfzeONu3Mo

TEDx Talks. (2018). *Collaboration in health care: The journey of an accidental expert?* [video]. YouTube. https://www.youtube.com/watch?v=qOV-5h0FpAo

The Joint Commission. (2010). *Advancing effective communication, cultural competence, and patient- and family-centered care.* https://www.jointcommission.org/-/media/tjc/documents/resources/patient-safety-topics/health-equity/aroadmapforhospitalsfinalversion727pdf.pdf?db=web&hash=AC3AC4BED1D973713C2CA6B2E5ACD01B

The Joint Commission. (2017, September 12). *Sentinel event alert.* https://e-handoff.com/wp-content/uploads/2017/09/Joint-Commision-Handoff-Communication-Alert.pdf

Thompson, C., & Stapley, S. (2011). Do educational interventions improve nurses' clinical decision making and judgement? A systematic review. *International Journal of Nursing Studies, 48*(7), 881–893. http://doi.org/10.1016/j.ijnurstu.2010.12.005

Tripathy, M. (2018). Assertiveness – A win-win approach to business communication. *IUP Journal of Soft Skills, 12*(2), 48-56. https://ssrn.com/abstract=3273251

Van Servellen, G. M. (2009). *Communication skills for the health care professional: Concepts, practice, and evidence.* Jones & Bartlett Publishers.

VitalSmarts Video. (2011, Mar 31). *Communication breakdown in healthcare.* [video]. YouTube. https://www.youtube.com/watch?v=BcC9YSTa8B8

Wang, Y., Wan, Q., Lin, F., Zhou, W., & Shang, S. (2017). Interventions to improve communication between nurses and physicians in the intensive care unit: A integrative literature review. *International Journal of Nursing Sciences, 5*, 81-88. http://doi.org/doi.org/10.1016/j.ijnss.2017.09.007

Weller, J., Boyd, M., & Cumin, D. (2014). Teams, tribes and patient safety: Overcoming barriers to effective teamwork in healthcare. *Postgraduate Medical Journal, 90*(1061), 149-154. http://doi.org/10.1136/postgradmedj-2012-131168

Westcott, M. R. (1968). *Toward a contemporary psychology of intuition: a historical, theoretical, and empirical inquiry.* Holt, Rinehart and Winston.

White, A. H. (2003). Clinical decision making among fourth-year nursing students: An interpretive study. *Journal of Nursing Education, 42*(3), 113-120. http://doi.org/10.3928/0148-4834-20030301-06

World Health Organization. (2010). *Framework for action on interprofessional education & collaborative practice.* Author.

Yang, Y., Lizardo, O., Wang, D., Dong, Y., Striegel, A. D., Hachen, D., & Chawla, N. V. (2016, May 24). *Gender differences in communication behaviors, spatial proximity patterns, and mobility habits.* https://arxiv.org/pdf/1607.06740.pdf

CHAPTER 4

Leadership in Nursing

Given the rapid and continual changes to the healthcare landscape, the integration of innovative technology, and an aging, complex patient population, the way in which care is delivered must be reimagined. In order to address these issues and improve the delivery of care, effective and efficient leadership is vital.

The current healthcare system requires visionary leaders to address the challenges of the current healthcare environment and to become an active player in healthcare reform. The landmark report by the Institute of Medicine (IOM, 2011), *The Future of Nursing, Leading Change, Advancing Health* focuses on transformation of nursing practice, nursing education, and nursing leadership. *The Future of Nursing, Leading Change, Advancing Health* can be found at the National Academies of Science website.

All nurses require leadership skills and competencies to in order to partner with physicians and other healthcare professionals, both within and outside of their institution. Nurses play a vital role in transforming healthcare, such as:

- Provision of safe, high quality, patient-centered care
- Primary care services
- Care delivery in the community
- Provision of seamless, coordinated care
- Accessible, affordable healthcare
- Engagement in health information technology (such as EMRs) (IOM, 2011)

In order for nurses to achieve these outcomes, nursing leadership must undergo a radical transformation. Health reform legislation signed by President Obama in 2010 includes a wide range of initiatives including the redesign of the healthcare delivery system. Many of the programs that have been created rely on interventions that inherent in registered nurses' scope of practice, such as care coordination and transitional care.

Being a leader, or a full partner in healthcare reform, means taking responsibility for recognizing problems or needs in the healthcare setting. Nurses at all levels of care must serve as strong advocates for patients and take the initiative to become involved with decision-making and offering suggestions on how to improve the delivery healthcare.

The delivery of high-quality nursing care is at risk during an era of critical transitions. The aging nursing workforce, retirement of nurse leaders, and the current and future nursing shortage requires strong nursing leadership. In order to achieve the vision of transforming the healthcare system, the profession must produce leaders throughout all areas the healthcare system. Leaders must be present at every level of care and across all settings. Nurses must be accountable for their contribution to providing high-quality care, while working collaboratively with leaders throughout the healthcare system (IOM, 2011).

The nursing workforce struggles with overextended, fatigued staff who are often disenchanted with the current work environment (Van Bogaert & Clarke, 2018). The healthcare system requires nurse leaders who are capable of creating a healthy work environment that instills trust, empowerment, support and encouragement, and a leadership style sustains nurses' health and well-being.

The IOM (2011) explains how an effective leadership style is essential in today's healthcare landscape, adding, "What is needed is a style of leadership that involves working with others as full partners in a context of mutual respect and collaboration" (p. 233). Leadership styles with a focus on respect and collaboration have been associated with improved patient outcomes, reduced medical errors, increased nurse retention and job satisfaction, improved teamwork, reduced lengths of hospital stay, and cost savings (IOM, 2011). Through effective nursing leadership, the nursing profession will continue to grow and evolve, and provide exceptional nursing care to patients who desperately need it.

Scope and Standards of Practice

As discussed in week 1, the Scope and Standards of Practice, developed by the American Nurses Association (ANA, 2015c), serves as a template for professional nursing practice for all registered nurses. Standard 11, Leadership, states, "The registered nurse leads within the professional practice setting and the profession" (ANA, 2010, p. 75). The following is a summary of the competencies of the Leadership standard:

- Contributes to the establishment of an environment that supports and maintains resect, trust, and dignity.
- Encourages innovation in practice and role performance to attain personal and professional plans, goals, and vision.
- Communicates to manage change and address conflict.
- Mentors colleagues for the advancement of nursing practice and the profession to enhance safe, quality health care.
- Retains accountability for delegated nursing care.
- Contributes to the evolution of the profession through participation in professional organizations.
- Influences policy to promote health (ANA, 2015, p. 75)

The goal of both formal and informal nursing leadership roles is to transform the healthcare system, where quality and safety are paramount.

Leadership Concepts and Definitions

Leadership: "a process whereby an individual influences a group of individuals to achieve a common goal" (Northouse, 2018, p. 5)

Note the following concepts within this definition:

- Leadership as a ***process***: leadership is not a characteristic or trait of an individual, but an event that occurs between a leader and follower or a leader and a group (Northouse, 2018)
- Leadership occurs in ***groups***: leadership occurs within groups, with people who have the same common goals or purpose as the leader (Northouse, 2018)
- Leadership has ***common goals***: leaders and followers have a common goal or purpose. Leaders work with followers to achieve selected goals (Northouse, 2018)
- Leadership involves ***influence***: leadership is focused on *how* the leader affects the followers, and the type of communication between the individuals (Ruben & Gigliotti, 2017)

Formal leaders: individuals who hold a formal leadership position, such as nurse manager.

Informal leaders: individuals who do not hold a position with formal authority, though are recognized as leaders, and have influence over their peers (Pielstick, 2000).

Informal leaders are higher performers with significant skill, they feel responsible for the functioning of their team, which they strengthen by exerting their influence by solving problems for colleagues who are in need (Downey, Parslow, & Smart, 2011).

Followers or subordinates: individuals who are being directed by a leader or manager.

Empowerment

Amundsen and Martinsen (2014) define empowerment as *giving* influence to others, rather than having influence *over*. The central characteristic of a leader who empowers others is one who supports and encourages autonomy. When a nurse manager *gives* influence to a staff nurse, the nurse has more power over decision-making, delegating, etc., which in turn leads to a more autonomous practice. Nurse leaders must use empowerment strategies in order for staff to have the freedom to make patient care decisions, especially in this challenging healthcare landscape (Spencer & McLaren, 2016).

Two types of empowerment:

- **Structural empowerment**: employees work in environments that have structure. When employees have access to opportunities, information, support, and necessary resources, they are able to be effective and achieve goals (Kanter, 1993)
- **Psychological empowerment**: fosters a proactive approach about achieving goals. Individuals learn how to cope within the workplace environment and have more control over their lives. In addition, individuals believe they are capable of influence and by understanding workplace/system processes they are able to engage in necessary behaviors to reach their goals (Zimmerman, 1995).

Empowerment is a way to encourage employees to work beyond the usual standards, supporting a flexible approach to completing tasks and reaching goals (Pearson & Moomaw, 2005). Working beyond usual standards has multiple meanings. For example, a nurse can take a more autonomous approach to practice, educating oneself on new evidence, making a suggestion about an outdated policy, or suggesting a team meeting. While these examples may be part of usual nursing practice, and expected of all nurses, nursing staff need the support of management to follow through with certain actions. Managers need to empower nurses in order for them to have a fully autonomous practice.

Chandler (1991) shares another viewpoint of empowerment as "enabling individuals to feel effective so that they can successfully execute their jobs" (p. 66). When managers empower their nursing staff, it helps improve their confidence in carrying out tasks as they see fit. A clinic nurse may decide to follow up with a patient who was recently hospitalized. The clinic manager or provider must provide a work environment where such decision-making, and freedom, can be made by

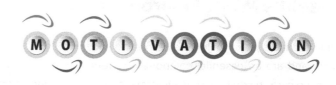

the nurse. When nurses have tight oversight from their managers, making autonomous decisions about care will be impeded, possibly leading to negative health outcomes.

Rao (2012) explains nursing empowerment as a condition where nurses have control over their practice when they successfully accomplish their goals, fulfill their responsibilities. Having control over one's practice is empowering, nurses have the authority, or influence, to complete their tasks as they see fit, which is akin to having an autonomous practice. When nurses are empowered by their managers, they have the resources, support, and encouragement to complete their tasks. When leaders empower their staff, they are also encouraging autonomous practice. See week 1 for a review on *Nursing Autonomy*.

Empowerment is foundational to interprofessional collaboration, and nursing practice as a whole, and it is associated with the following outcomes:

- Increased job satisfaction
- Increased trust within the organization
- Improved effectiveness within the nursing unit
- Positive coworker relationships (Read & Laschinger, 2015; Regan, Laschinger, & Wong, 2015)

Working in today's healthcare environment has forced leaders to improvise, creating ways to prepare themselves, and their team, to cope with workplace stressors, such as workplace bullying. Leaders can focus their efforts on strengthening empowerment, both structural and psychological, within the workplace to meet create a positive and productive environment.

Nurses as leaders at all levels, across all settings

Strong nursing leadership is required in all settings, from the bedside, to the community nurse, nurse managers, director of nursing, members of nursing organizations, nurse researchers, school nurses, etc. Nurses must exercise their leadership competencies collaboratively in all settings, such as hospitals, communities, schools, businesses, boards, the political arena, and more. All nurses must take responsibility for their professional growth by developing leadership skills and competencies in their area of specialty (IOM, 2011). Below are some examples of effective leadership from bedside to boardroom:

- Awareness of the need to advocate, mediate, collaborate
- Link actions to quality care
- Nurses' technical ability to deliver care in a safe and effective manner
- Improving work processes at the bedside/frontline
- Creating or offering new evidence for practice
- Collaborate with policy makers
- Craft policy and legislation that allows nurses to work to their fullest capacity
- Lead nursing education/curriculum changes to prepare the nursing workforce to meet the needs of a complex healthcare environment
- Serve on institutional and policy-making boards where critical decisions affecting patients are made
- Autonomous practice in community health settings
- Assertiveness, to have a strong voice in advocating for patients and their families (IOM, 2011)

Healthy Work Environments

Nurse leaders play a major role in creating and maintaining healthy work environments (HWE). HWEs foster excellence in patient care and are an essential component to reversing the current nursing shortage and providing safe, quality, compassionate nursing care. In addition, HWEs improve nurses' well-being and their perception of feeling fulfilled at work (American Association of Critical Care Nurses [AACN], 2016).

Unhealthy work environments lead to:

- Medical errors
- Ineffective delivery of care
- Conflict and stress among health care professionals (AACN, 2016)

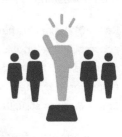

Today's work environments demand increased attention to these negative consequences. In order to improve practice environments and nursing practice itself, nurse leaders must be positioned within their organization to have the power to inform and influence decision-making (AACN, 2016). Nurse leaders, such as nurse managers, must have the following core competencies and skills to create HWE environments:

- self-knowledge
- strategic vision
- risk-taking
- creativity
- interpersonal and communication effectiveness
- inspiration (Wong & Giallonardo, 2013)
- team builders
- agents for positive change
- role models for collaboration
- committed to service (Shirey, 2009).

AACN's (2016) Healthy Work Environment Model has developed six evidence-based standards that can improve or maintain a healthy work environment:

1. **Skilled communication**

   - Nurses must be as proficient in communication skills as they are in clinical skills

2. **True collaboration**

   - Nurses must be relentless in pursuing and fostering true collaboration

3. **Effective decision-making**

   - Nurses must be valued and committed partners in making policy, directing and evaluating clinical care, and leading organizational operations

4. **Appropriate staffing**

   - Staffing must ensure the effective match between patient needs and nurse competencies

5. **Meaningful recognition**

   - Nurses must be recognized and must recognize others for the value each brings to the work of the organization

6. **Authentic leadership**

   - Nurse leaders must fully embrace the imperative of a healthy work environment, authentically live it, and engage others in its achievement

The critical elements needed to transform and maintain HWE requires the authentic leader to perform as follows:

- share an understanding of the requirements and dynamics for providing direct patient care
- generate an enthusiasm for meeting goals (including a HWE)
- role model all six HWE standards
- nurse leaders and team members objectively evaluate the impact of the leadership processes and decision-making in relation to HWE goals

While formal leaders, such as nurse managers, are easily positioned to inform practice though collaboration with other executives and formal leaders in nursing administration, bedside or staff nurses also play a major role with incorporating all six standards into practice. Communication, collaboration, effective decision-making, and leadership skills are integrated into all nursing roles. Nurses owe it to their patients, the nursing profession, and society to advance quality care and improve the overall health of the population.

Mentoring

According to the ANA (2015c) and the IOM (2010), all nurses are leaders, and one of the expectations of being a formal or informal leader is to mentor one's peers. Mentoring is critical for advancement of nursing practice and the nursing profession as a whole, because when nurses mentor, counsel, or support their peers, the quality of nursing care is improved. Some example of mentoring can include the following:

- Educate how to perform a new skill
- How to problem-solve a complex patient concern
- Share advice on time management
- Encourage a peer when overwhelmed
- Reassurance about abilities or skills
- Advise on career goals, share guidance/suggestions

See week 2 resource, *Professional Development Plan*, for more information about mentoring.

Partnerships

Participating in community partnerships is essential for advancing the profession and transforming healthcare. The IOM (2010) discusses the importance of nurses developing partnerships with agencies or stakeholders within the community. For example, a nurse could become a member of an ethics committee at a local nursing home or create a relationship with a local food bank or soup kitchen to assist with discharge planning. Sharing knowledge from one's current role and setting with community stakeholders advances everyone's knowledge about each other's needs, available services, all leading to improving the ability to better serve patient needs.

When nurses are knowledgeable about their community, and the care and services available to their patients, they are taking important steps towards transforming healthcare. Partnerships are indispensable for reaching the overarching goal of quality healthcare for all.

Nurses as "full partners"

In order for nurses to be a full partner in transforming healthcare, all nurses must acquire leadership skills and competencies and collaborate with other healthcare professionals and organizations. Some examples of being a full partner in patient care settings includes the following activities:

- taking responsibility for identifying problems and areas of waste
- devising and implementing a plan for improvement
- tracking improvement over time
- maintain a focus on short- and long-term goals; making necessary adjustments to realize established goals (IOM, 2011)

Considering the amount of time nurses spend with patients, compared to other disciplines, nurses are in a strategic position to identify problem areas, whether it's due to a patient need or concern, or a policy, procedure, or process that impedes care. Both formal and informal leaders need to share ideas for improvement and become vested in finding solutions.

Nurses can improve workflow, improve safety of the work environment or learning new ways of team communication by taking the imitative to seek out new knowledge from the literature (such as library databases). While formal leaders, such as a nurse manager or nurse executive, may have more power to follow through with policy changes, informal leaders are integral to the process of identifying problems and offering solutions.

Nurse leaders also need to have an active voice with health policy. Healthcare reform requires nurses to take an active role with implementation of political activism efforts. Nurses can serve on advisory committees, commissions, hospital committees, and boards where policies are created or amended to advance healthcare (IOM, 2011). Participation in a committee within one's organization takes time and effort, though brings many rewards, both personally and professionally. Consider creating a goal in your professional development plan that can impact health policy. Some examples include advocating for safe staffing at hospitals or ethical treatment at end of life.

Sigma Theta Tau International

The need for excellent leadership is essential in today's rapidly changing, complex healthcare environment. Sigma Theta Tau International (STTI) is a global professional nursing organization with the mission of advancing healthcare and celebrate nursing excellence in scholarship, leadership, and service. STTI advocates for strong, positive leadership throughout the nursing profession in order to advance health (Vlasich, 2017).

STTI's role is to develop leadership knowledge, skills and abilities for nurses globally. STTI believes leadership develops throughout one's career, it is a journey of lifelong learning, with mentoring as the cornerstone of one's leadership philosophy (Vlasich, 2017).

STTI (2020b) offers membership to students who are working towards a baccalaureate degree where nurses are developing leadership knowledge, skills and abilities. In order to become a member of STTI, students must meet the following criteria:

- Completed half of the nursing curriculum.
- Achieve academic excellence:
  - For universities/institutions of higher education that use a 4.0 grade point average system to measure academic achievement, baccalaureate students must have a cumulative grade point average (GPA) of at least 3.0.
- Students must rank in the top 35% of the graduating class
- Meet the expectation of academic integrity (STTI, 2020b)

STTI also provides leadership grants to assist nurses with membership fees and travel to Sigma events (STTI, 2020a).

For more additional information about membership visit the STTI website.

Leadership Theory and Leadership Styles

Leadership theories and styles focus on a wide variety of ways to lead others, such as an emphasis on serving others, creating relationships, having power and control over others, or working together to reach goals. This section will review the major concepts of leadership styles and some of the most common leadership theories.

Leadership styles are categorized based on human relationships or task completion (Cummings et al., 2018). The following is a brief overview of current leadership styles:

> **Feminine leadership style** emphasizes a *power with* approach (Burns, 1978). Sindell and Shamberger (2016) explain the following feminine expressions:

- listen for the emotional context and connection
- listens to others in order to sympathize with their emotions
- consoles, supports
- shares an emotional reaction
- supportive in areas of employee progress and development

> **Masculine leadership style** emphasizes a *power over* approach (Burns, 1978). Sindell and Shamberger (2016) explain the following masculine expressions:

- listens for content and clarity
- ignores other's emotions
- does not express one's emotions

Leadership Theories and Styles

Goh, Ang, and Della (2018) discuss the importance of examining one's professional leadership style and its impact on peers, employees, goal attainment, and outcomes. Self-reflection could motivate one to find a leadership theory or style that can bring about overall improved outcomes.

One leadership theory or style is not necessarily better than the other. Each theory or style has its strengths and weaknesses, and depending on one's perspective, goals, work setting, task, and even gender*, some leadership styles may produce better patient outcomes or higher job satisfaction.

Table 1 below complies a brief list of the some of the most commonly used leadership theories and styles:

Table 1: Leadership Theories

Transformational leadership	Transformational leadership has a positive and direct association with the level of organization commitment and retention of staff. Leadership qualities include charisma or non-verbal influence, inspirational motivation, intellectual stimulation, and individualized consideration. These leaders are admired, trusted, and respected. Leadership qualities have a significant impact on patient outcomes due to how well leaders inspire and motivate staff. Followers of this leadership style are more involved in their organization and put more effort in their work (Al, Galdas, & Watson, 2018)
Transactional leadership	Transactional leaders use a task-focused approach, whereby managers will motivate employees using punishment and reward. These leaders have the potential to improve job satisfaction, though overall, this style is associated with reduced empowerment and poorer health and well-being of staff (Cummings et al., 2018)
Authentic leadership	Authentic leadership is a relational leadership style that inspires staff performance and organizational outcomes. These leaders promote healthy work environments. Authentic leadership results in trust in the manager, job satisfaction, structural empowerment, positive work engagement, and work group relationships (Alilyyani, Wong, & Cummings. 2018)
Servant leadership	Servant leadership focuses on benevolent service to others. The servant leader puts employees first and promotes their well-being and growth and considers the interests of customers and the community. Servant leaders are role models of considerate treatment of others and help others in their development and growth. Servant leadership is akin to how nurses provide patient care, as nurses main focus is on their patients' overall well-being and satisfaction (Neubert, Hunter, & Tolentino, 2016)
Path-goal leadership	Path-goal leadership motivates team members to accomplish designated goals by emphasizing the relationship between the leader, the follower, and the tasks. Path-goal leaders reward employees for meeting goals, leading to improved job satisfaction. This leadership defines goals, clarifies the path, removes obstacles, and provides support for task completion. Path-goal leaders understand the needs of the employee and shift their leadership style as necessary to motivate their employees to complete the task (Bickle, 2017)
Situational leadership	Situational leaders judge the response by the follower based on their ability and willingness to complete the task. The leader responds with one of four quadrants: • **Telling:** high task/low relationship (leader in command, situation with one correct response) • **Selling:** high task/high relationship (leader has most controls, assists subordinates with confidence to complete task) • **Participating:** high relationship/low task (leader and subordinate share decision-making) • **Delegating:** low task/low relationship (leader trusts subordinate's ability to take full responsibility for making decisions/completing task) (Hershey & Blanchard, 1977) Communication tools can be applied to each of the four quadrants to create an environment where communication is open, concerns and thoughts are expressed freely, and mutual understanding can become the standard within the organization. The primary consideration for a situational leader is communication and ensuring communication is clear and in partnership with the follower. By adjusting the leadership style to meet the followers' needs, the follower grows and becomes more capable of completing the required tasks (Wright, 2017)
Theory X	Theory X leaders assume that employees will avoid work if possible, and they are inherently lazy and dislike work. Theory X leaders closely supervise employees (micromanage) and rely heavily on threat and intimidation to stimulate productivity. These leaders provide clear expectations of the work they expect to be done, how it should be done, and how long it should take (Hattangadi, 2015)
Theory Y	Theory Y leaders assume employees will practice self-direction in achieving the goals and objectives of the organization and they are committed to those objectives. These leaders offer guidance and promote autonomy to their followers. Theory Y leaders engage their employees in decision-making processes to inspire motivation and creativity (Hattangadi, 2015)

Authoritarian	Authoritarian leaders do not develop relationships with their employees. This type of leadership meets goals through making demands, instituting punishments, regulations, rules and orders. These leaders are in full charge of decision-and rule-making and problem-solving. Followers must adhere to all the leader's instructions without input and cannot question an order. Authoritarian leaders make all the decisions without employee involvement (Greenfield, 2007) Authoritarian leadership can be an asset in situations where an urgent task must be completed in a timely manner. The authoritarian leader's discipline and structure is essential in these situations (Wiesenthal, Kalpna, McDowell, & Radin, 2015)
Democratic	Democratic leaders facilitate collective decision-making, encouraging freedom and autonomy among team members. These leaders empower, support, and encourage their followers to make independent choices, thus supporting independent autonomous decision-making. Some of the core leadership traits include cooperation, active participation, accountability, and delegation of responsibilities and tasks (Avolio, Walumbwa, & Weber, 2009) Since democratic leaders encourage autonomous and collective decision-making, the risk for role ambiguity and longer task completion can occur (Rahbi, Khalid, & Khan, 2017)
Laissez-faire	Laissez-faire leadership is defined as "… the avoidance or absence of leadership and is, by definition, the most inactive and most ineffective according to almost all research on the style (Bass & Avolio, 1994) Laissez-faire leadership has been found to be the root cause of workplace role stress, which has the potential to negatively impact job satisfaction and work effectiveness (especially for those subordinates who are in need of active leadership) (Skogstad, Hetland, Glasø, & Einarsen, 2014)
Management by Walking Around also called **Leading by Walking Around**	**Benefits:** • Observes team members interacting with patients and with each other • Shows the team members the leader is vested in the team and interested their work • Ability to evaluate unit processes • Opportunity to evaluate the quality of work • Demonstrates interest in daily operations • Leaders can ascertain how well a unit functions through purposeful listening (Frandsen, 2014)

Leadership Characteristics

Burke, Flanagan, Ditomassi, and Hickey (2018) discusses nurse retention as an essential part of patient care delivery system. Thus, all nurse leaders must concentrate on creating ways to attract and retain nurses. Leadership characteristics identified by Burke et al. (2018) reflect transformational leadership, known to enhance job satisfaction. Qualities of exemplary nurse leaders include the following:

• Passion
• Optimism
• Personal connection
• Role modeling
• Leadership mentoring
• Presence
• Availability

Burke et al. (2018) found registered nurses found the following NM behaviors positively impacted their job satisfaction:

• Empowerment and Reflective Practice: a focus on enhancing nurse autonomy
• Passion and Vision: the quest for excellence
• Visibility: promotes interpersonal connections leading to a safe and caring environment
• High Expectations and Professional Behaviors: Appreciate and value the role modeled by NMs

Leading Four Generations of Nurses

Frandsen (2014) discusses the generational divide in today's workplace, and how nurses from four generations are working together for the first time in history. Frandsen (2014) describes the characteristics of each generation:

Silent Generation or Veterans or Traditionalists (1925-1945)

- Likely the most disciplined employee, loyal
- Seek approval from their employers, a traditional work ethic
- Often have a lifetime career with one employer or one field of work
- Respect for authority

Baby Boomer (1946-1964)

- Optimistic, competitive, focus on personal accomplishment.
- Work hard, often stressed, focus on achievement, seek self-improvement,
- Complain though accept problems
- In conflict with younger generations who do not share their values
- Primary focus is on work, resulting in a higher susceptibility to burnout and stress-related illness

Generation X (1965-1980)

- Many were "latch-key" children, resulting in a sense of independence that causes resentment when peers supervise their work
- Question authority
- Expect immediate results
- Committed to their team and manager
- Loyalty resides more with their peers and supervisor than with the organization

Generation Y or Echo Boomers or Millennial (1981-2000)

- Team-oriented
- Works well in groups
- Multitasks
- Willingness to work hard
- Expects structure in the workplace
- Respects positions and titles, seeks a satisfying relationship with managers
- Seeks out continuing education, professional development
- Desire to establish a relationship with their manager may cause conflict with Gen Xers who choose a hands-off approach

In order to understand peers or followers, leaders must reflect on their own generational characteristics (André, 2018).

References

AI, Y. M., Galdas, P., & Watson, R. (2018). Leadership style and organisational commitment among nursing staff in Saudi Arabia. *Journal of Nursing Management, 26*(5), 531–539. http://doi.org/10.1111/jonm.12578

Alilyyani, B., Wong, C. A., & Cummings, G. (2018). Antecedents, mediators, and outcomes of authentic leadership in healthcare: A systematic review. *International Journal of Nursing Studies.* http://doi.org/10.1016/j.ijnurstu.2018.04.001

American Association of Critical-Care Nurses. (2016). *AACN standards for establishing and sustaining healthy work environments. A journey to excellence.* (2nd ed.). Author

American Nurses Association. (2015). *Scope and standards of practice* (3rd ed.). Author.

Amundsen, S., & Martinsen, Ø. L. (2014). Empowering leadership: Construct clarification, conceptualization, and validation of a new scale. *Leadership Quarterly, 25,* 487-511. http://doi.org/10.1016/j.leaqua.2013.11.009

André, S. (2018). Embracing generational diversity: Reducing and managing workplace conflict. *ORNAC Journal, 36*(4), 13–35. http://doi.org/10.1310/hpj4807-537

Avolio, B., Walumbwa, F. & Weber, T.J. (2009). Leadership: Current theories, research and future directions. *Annual Review of Psychology, 60,* 421-49. http://doi.org/10.1146/annurev.psych.60.110707.163621

Bass, B. M., & Avolio, B. J. (1994). *Improving organizational effectiveness through transformational leadership.* Sage Publications.

Bickle, J. T. (2017). Developing remote training consultants as leaders-dialogic/network application of path-goal leadership theory in leadership development. *Performance Improvement, 56*(9), 32-39. http://doi.org/10.1002/pfi.21738

Burke, D., Flanagan, J., Ditomassi, M., & Hickey, P. A. (2018). Characteristics of nurse directors that contribute to registered nurse satisfaction. *Journal of Nursing Administration, 47*(4), S12-S18. http://doi.org/10.1097/NNA.0000000000000468

Burns, J. (1978). *Leadership.* Harper & Row.

Chandler, G. E. (1991). Creating an environment to empower nurses. *Nursing Management, 22*(8), 20–23. https://journals.lww.com/nursingmanagement/citation/1991/08000/creating_an_environment_to_empower_nurses.6.aspx

Cummings, G. G., MacGregor, T., Davey, M., Lee, H., Wong, C. A., Lo, E., Muise, M., & Stafford, E. (2018). Leadership styles and outcome patterns for the nursing workforce and work environment: A systematic review. *International Journal of Nursing Studies, 85,* 19–60. http://doi.org/10.1016/j.ijnurstu.2018.04.016

Downey, M., Parslow, S., & Smart, M. (2011). The hidden treasure in nursing leadership: Informal leaders. *Journal of Nursing Management, 19*(4), 517-521. http://doi.org/10.1111/j.1365-2834.2011.01253.x

Frandsen, B. (2014). *Nursing leadership management & leadership styles.* https://www.aanac.org/docs/white-papers/2013-nursing-leadership—management-leadership-styles.pdf?sfvrsn=4

Goh, A. M. J., Ang, S. Y., & Della, P. R. (2018). Leadership style of nurse managers as perceived by registered nurses: A cross-sectional survey. *Proceedings of Singapore Healthcare, 27*(3), 205-210. http://doi.org/10/2.1011707/120510810757851177541 2742

Greenfield, D. (2007). The enactment of dynamic leadership. *Leadership in Health Services, 20*(3), 159-68. http://doi.org/10.1108/17511870710764014

Hattangadi, V. (2015). Theory X & theory Y. *International Journal of Recent Research Aspects, 2*(4), 20–21.

Hershey, P. & Blanchard, K. (1977). *Management of organizational behavior: Leading human resources.* (3rd ed.). Prentice Hall

Institute of Medicine. (2010). *The future of nursing: Leading change advancing health.* National Academies Press.

Kanter, R. M. (1977). *Men and women of the corporation.* Basic Books.

Kanter, R. M. (1979). Power failure in management circuits. *Classics of Organization Theory,* 342-351.

McCay, R., Lyles, A. A., & Larkey, L. (2018). Nurse leadership style, nurse satisfaction, and patient satisfaction: A systematic review. *Journal of Nursing Care Quality, 33*(4), 361-367. http://doi.org/10.1097/NCQ.0000000000000317

Neubert, M. J., Hunter, E. M., & Tolentino, R. C. (2016). A servant leader and their stakeholders: When does organizational structure enhance a leader's influence? *The Leadership Quarterly,* (6), 1-15. http://dx.doi.org/10.1016/j.leaqua.2016.05.005

Northouse, P. G. (2018). *Leadership: Theory and practice* (8th ed.). Sage Publications.

Pearson, L. C., & Moomaw, W. (2005). The relationship between teacher autonomy and stress, work satisfaction, empowerment, and professionalism. *Educational Research Quarterly, 29*(1), 38-54.

Pielstick, C. D. (2000). Formal vs. informal leading: A comparative analysis. *Journal of Leadership & Organizational Studies, 7*(3), 99-114. http://doi.org/10.1177/107179190000700307

Rahbi, D. A., Khalid, K., & Khan, M. (2017). The effects of leadership styles on team motivation. *Academy of Strategic Management Journal, 16*(2), 1-14. https://www.abacademies.org/articles/The-effects-of-leadership-styles-1939-6104-16-3-113.pdf

Rao A. (2012). The contemporary construction of nurse empowerment. *Journal of Nursing Scholarship, 44*(4), 396–402. http://doi.org/10.1111/j.1547-5069.2012.01473.x

Read, E. A., & Laschinger, H. K. S. (2015). The influence of authentic leadership and empowerment on nurses' relational social capital, mental health and job satisfaction over the first year of practice. *Journal of Advanced Nursing, 71*(1), 1611- 1623. http://doi.org/10.1111/jan.12625

Regan, S., Laschinger, H. K. S., & Wong, C. A. (2015). The influence of empowerment, authentic leadership, and professional practice environments on nurses' perceived interprofessional collaboration. *Journal of Nursing Management, 24*(1), E54- E61. http://doi.org/10.1111/jonm.12288

Ruben, B. D., & Gigliotti, R. A. (2017). Communication: Sine qua non of organizational leadership theory and practice. *International Journal of Business Communication, 54*(1), 12-30. http://doi.org/10.1177/2329488416675447

Shirey, M. R. (2009). Authentic leadership, organizational culture, and healthy work environments. *Critical Care Nursing Quarterly, 32*(3), 189-198. http://doi.org/10.1097/CNQ.0b013e3181ab91db

Sigma Theta Tau International. (2020a). Leadership education grants. https://www.sigmanursing.org/why-sigma/sigma-foundation-for-nursing/what-we-do/leadership-education-grantsmembership-criteria

Sigma Theta Tau International. (2020b). Student membership criteria. https://www.sigmanursing.org/why-sigma/sigma-membership/apply-now/student-membership-criteria

Sindell, T., & Shamberger, S. (2016). Beyond gender: Changing the leadership conversation. *People & Strategy, 39*(3), 32–35.

Skogstad, A., Hetland, J., Glasø, L., & Einarsen, S. (2014). Is avoidant leadership a root cause of subordinate stress? Longitudinal relationships between laissez-faire leadership and role ambiguity. *Work & Stress, 28*(4), 323–341. http://doi.org/10.1080/02678373.2014.957362

Spencer, C., & McLaren, S. (2016). Empowerment in nurse leader groups in middle management: A quantitative comparative investigation. *Journal of Clinical Nursing, 26*(1-2), 266-279. http://doi.org/10.1111/jocn.13426

Van Bogaert, P., & Clarke, S., (2018). *The organizational context of nursing practice: Concepts evidence, and interventions for improvement.* Springer.

Vlasich, C. (2017). The quest for excellent leadership. *Journal of Nursing Management, 25*(5), 327–328. http://doi.org/10.1111/jonm.12497

Wiesenthal, A. M., Kalpna, J., McDowell, T., & Radin, J. (2015). The new physician leaders: Leadership for a dynamic health. *The New England Journal of Medicine*, 1-3.

Wong, C. A., & M. Giallonardo, L. (2013). Authentic leadership and nurse-assessed adverse patient outcomes. *Journal of Nursing Management, 21*(5), 740-752. http://doi.org/10.1111/jonm.12075

Wright, E. S. (2017). Dialogic development in the situational leadership style. *Performance Improvement, 56*(9), 27–31. http://doi.org/10.1002/pfi.21733

Zimmerman, M. A. (1995). Psychological empowerment: Issues and illustrations. *American Journal of Community Psychology, 23*(5), 581-599.

CHAPTER 5

Nursing Theory

The overarching goal of nursing theories is to define what nursing is, how and why nurses do what they do, and to provide a framework for making decisions. This chapter will review the different levels of nursing theory, evaluate the assumptions made by different nursing theorists, and learn how to apply nursing theory to practice situations.

The primary purpose of creating nursing theories are to guide nursing practice. Nursing theory can be integrated into any nursing setting, such as a hospital or community-based clinic. Theories can also be integrated into specific clinical settings, such as labor and delivery. Theories are beneficial to nursing practice in numerous ways. When nurses incorporate theory into personal nursing practice, it allows for creativity and implementation of innovative interventions. Many nursing behaviors are based on theory, such as caring and patient education. Nursing theory helps nurses organize their care

The first step to understanding nursing theory is to understand the attributes of a theory. The list below shares the attributes found in every nursing theory, and while uncommon, some theories may not share assumptions depending on the year they were created.

Theory Attributes

Concept

- Building block of all theories
- Components of every theory
- Variables that are tested during research (Mintz-Binder, 2019)
- For example, anxiety is a concept, which may or may not be easy to identify. Though anxiety can be identified through behaviors or symptoms. A patient who has anxiety may exhibit rapid breathing, palpitations, or irritation.

Theory

- Weaves together concepts to describe their relationships with each other
- Explains the relationships among the concepts
- Explains how these relationships interrelate with each other (Mintz-Binder, 2019)

Model

- A diagram of concepts and their relationship with each other (Morse, 2017)

Theoretical Framework

- Used for conducting research or the underpinning of policy
- Represents what the researcher thinks will happen in the study based on the chosen theory
- Way of organizing the concepts (called variables in research) and their relationship with each other
- By creating a model, a framework visually illustrates how a research study will be conducted, based on the theory (Morse, 2017)

Assumption

- Premise without proof
- Something usually unspoken, believed to be the truth, though no hard proof
- Something taken for granted (Morse, 2017)

Proposition

- Statements that link the concepts together
- Beliefs about the theory shared as statements
- Explains the reasoning for the relationship between the concepts (Mintz-Binder, 2019)

Metaparadigm

- A process by which an academic discipline communicates its fundamental characteristics
- All nursing theories address each concept by defining the concept and applying it to concepts or tenets of the theory
- Nursing metaparadigm consists of four concepts:

  1. **Person:** The focus of nursing care

     - Example: Watson's Theory of Human Caring views the patient holistically, while Johnson's Behavioral System model views the person through a lens of seven different subsystems

  2. **Health:** Depending on the theorist, health and illness can be perceived as two separate constructs (or concepts) or health and illness is viewed as a continuum (changes slowly over time)

     - Example: King's Theory of Goal Attainment views health a functional state throughout a person's life (a continuum), while Neuman's Systems model views health and illness as two separate constructs

  3. **Nursing:** A process whereby nurses provide care. The process changes based on the theorist.

     - Example: Watson's Theory of Human Caring views nursing as provision of care using the 10 carative factors whereas Orem's Self-Care Deficit theory where nurses' focus of care is assisting patients to meet their self-care needs

  4. **Environment:** the person's environment within a global context (Mintz-Binder, 2019)

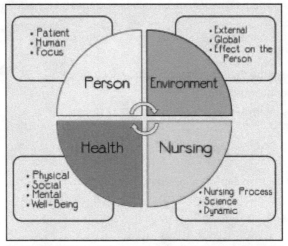

(Karp, 2019)

Two Types of Nursing Theories

Nursing theories are differentiated between grand and middle-range theories. Theories are placed in one of the two categories based on the following:

- Relevancy to nursing situations and clinical settings
- Broad or narrow focus
- Abstract or concrete concepts
- Detailed descriptions (Mintz-Binder, 2019)

Grand Theory

- Broad focus
- Abstract concepts and descriptions
- Represents ideas and thinking about nursing as a whole (Mintz-Binder, 2019)
    - Examples:
        - Johnson's Behavioral System's model
        - Roy's Adaptation model
        - Rogers' Science of Unitary Beings
        - Orem's Self-Care Deficit Nursing theory
        - Watson's Theory of Human Caring

Middle-Range Theory

- Created in the 1990s
- Narrower focus, more concrete, specific
- Focused on a clinical specialty
- Created with less depth and detail than grand theories (Mintz-Binder, 2019)
    - Examples:
        - Kolcaba's Comfort theory
        - Pender's Health Promotion model
        - Swanson's Theory of Caring
        - Leininger's Culture Care Theory
        - Peplau's Theory of Interpersonal Relations

Nursing Theory and Research

The following is a basic introduction to research and the use of a theoretical framework using nursing theory. Nursing research studies are often designed using a theoretical framework. This means a nursing theory (that aligns with the focus of the study) is chosen as the theoretical framework. Research studies are conducted to offer new knowledge and generate new evidence-based interventions.

For example, Meleis' Transitions Theory is focused on the different transitions that occur in people's lives, how people are supported during a role change and how they understand the transition (Meleis, Sawyer, Im, Messias, & Schumacher, 2000). A researcher who wants to understand the transition for a woman giving birth, becoming a mother for the first time, may use Meleis' Transitions Theory as a theoretical framework to guide the design of the study.

Research studies may create models to design the study. The model incorporates all the major concepts of the theory. The major concepts of each theory are the core elements of each theory.

Nursing Theory for Policy Creation

As discussed above, nursing theorists create new knowledge by designing and testing theories through conducting research. The knowledge gleaned from research is used to create policies that provide nursing practice with best practice standards. Since there are many types of nursing theories and models, with a varying focus, different types of policies can be created based on many different nursing theories. The examples below demonstrate how knowledge gathered from nursing theory can guide policy creation, and in turn, positively impact nursing practice:

- **Pain management:** the Acute Pain Management Theory offers guidance on the role of the patient participating in pain management, such balancing the side effects of pain medication and reduced pain.
- **Staffing:** when nurse-patient ratios are based on acuity, the Self-care Deficit Nursing Theory helps nurses determine the number of nurses needed for staffing based on patients' level of self-care. More than one theory can be used to assist with creating a ratio.
- **Health Promotion:** concepts of Pender's Health Promotion Model offer knowledge about patient behaviors that are associated with engaging in health-promotion activities.

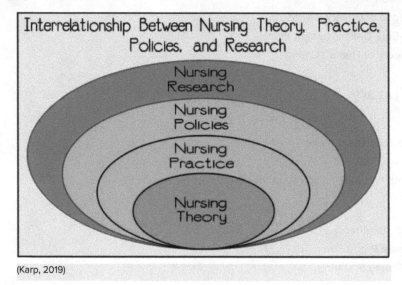

Interrelationship Between Nursing Theory, Practice, Policies, and Research

Nursing Research
Nursing Policies
Nursing Practice
Nursing Theory

(Karp, 2019)

Nursing Theory and Personal Nursing Philosophy

Nursing theory is a vital component of nursing practice and can positively impact practice especially when part of a nurse's personal nursing philosophy. Nurses can choose one or more theories that align to their practice and add additional statements about the theory to their nursing philosophy. For example, nurses working hospice may choose Watson's Theory of Human Caring. Applying the caritas #4, "Developing and sustaining a helping-trusting, authentic, caring relationship" (Watson, 2008, p. 31) can help the nurse instill certain attributes during interactions with the patient and family.

References

Meleis, A. I., Sawyer, L. M., Im, E. O., Messias, D. K. H., & Schumacher, K. (2000). Experiencing transitions: An emerging middle-range theory. *Advances in Nursing Science, 23*(1), 12-28. http://doi.org/10.1097/00012272-200009000-00006

Mintz-Binder, R. (2019). The connection between nursing theory and practice. *Nursing Made Incredibly Easy, 17*(1). http://doi.org/10.1097/01.NME.0000549615.05397.55

Morse, J. M. (2017). *Analyzing and conceptualizing the theoretical foundations of nursing.* Springer Publishing Company.

Watson, J. (2008). *Nursing: The philosophy and science of caring.* (Revised ed.). University Press of Colorado

CHAPTER 6

Professional Organizations

Professional organizations were created as a platform for nurses to advocate for the profession, support nurses' rights, and ensure quality healthcare for consumers (Echevarria, 2018). Members of professional organizations can advocate locally, state-wide, nationally, and globally to support issues that impact the nursing profession and healthcare as a whole.

Nurses can choose from hundreds of professional organizations to advocate for the profession and attain a wide variety of membership benefits. For a list of national, state, and international professional organizations, visit https://nurse.org/orgs.shtml.

See week 1 resources under "Professional Nursing" for a review of accrediting and other professional organizations (ANA, NLN, AACN, and NCSBN).

Benefits of Membership

Membership within professional organizations offers nurses infinite opportunities to make a significant impact with advancing the profession, professional growth, and the healthcare system. Echevarria (2018) shares some additional ways to get involved:

- Advocate for healthcare consumers' rights, health, and safety
- Influence healthcare delivery by participating in, promoting, and using evidence-based knowledge and research findings to guide practice and decision-making
- Promote the ethical principles of research
- Identify barriers and opportunities to improve healthcare safety, equitability, and efficiency
- Critically review policies, procedures, and guidelines to improve quality
- Influence organizational policies and procedures to guide practice and promote interprofessional, evidence-based practices
- Advocate for resources that promote and support nursing practice

*See week 2 resources under "Professional Development Plan" for a full discussion about the role of mentoring and networking in professional nursing.

In addition to serving the profession and improving the healthcare system, membership offers nurses a multitude of professional benefits. Some benefits also include:

- Continuing education
- Specialty certification
- Best practices for nursing care
- Promote the rights of nurses
- Synchronous and asynchronous webinars
- Face-to-face seminars
- Journal access
- Career resources, job boards
- Conference engagements and opportunities (Echevarria, 2018)
- Discount on conference and certification registration fees
- Personal benefits, such as discounts on car rental, life insurance, professional liability insurance, and more

Nursing Scope and Standards of Practice

Nurses who take advantage of the activities offered by professional organizations meet the competencies for Standard 12, Education, in the ANA (2015c) Nursing Scope and Standards of Practice. For example, attending conferences offer nurses an opportunity to share their research and knowledge through podium and poster presentations. Participation in professional development opportunities, such as listening to a webinar or reading a nursing journal meets the following competencies for Standard 12:

- Shares educational findings, experiences, and ideas with peers.
- Demonstrates a commitment to lifelong learning through self-reflection and inquiry for learning and personal growth.
- Maintains a professional portfolio that provides evidence of individual competence and lifelong learning (ANA, 2015c, p. 76)

The following six values of membership in professional organizations aligns with the American Nurses Association (ANA, 2015c) *Nursing Scope and Standards of Practice*:

- Advocacy
- Professional development
- Service to the profession
- Career growth
- Mentoring*
- Networking*

Code of Ethics

Provision 9 of the ANA (2015a) *Code of Ethics* includes a requirement about advocacy efforts. Advocacy is fundamental to nursing practice, and through membership and participation in professional organizations, nurses can fulfill the following provision: "The profession of nursing, collectively through its professional organizations, must articulate nursing values, maintain the integrity of the profession, and integrate principles of social justice into nursing and health policy" (ANA, 2015a, p. 151).

How to Get Involved

The New York State Nurses Association (NYSNA) sponsors the annual Lobby Day in Albany, NY. Thousands of nurses gather each year to organize their efforts and meet with legislators to share their position on the current bills in the house or senate. For information about Lobby Day, visit NYSNA's website. One of the hotly debated topics nurses have discussed with legislators for years (almost 10 years) at Lobby Day is the Safe Staffing for Quality Care Act. A summary of the bill with the proposed nurse-patient ratios can be found at the NYSNA website and the actual bill can be viewed at the NY State Assembly website.

The ANA also has an annual Lobby Day Lobby Day in Washington D.C. Hundreds of nurses gather at Capitol Hill to meet with federal lawmakers to discuss major health issues, such as workplace violence, Title VIII Nursing Workforce Reauthorization Act of 2019, Home Health Care Planning Improvement Act of 2019 and more (Capitol Beat, 2019). For information about Lobby Day, visit ANA's website.

Participating in professional organization activities gives nurses an opportunity to give back to the profession. Echevarria (2018) shares a number of volunteer options for nurses:

- Participate on committees and task forces
- Hold a board position (see NOBC narrative below)
- Assist with organization-sponsored conferences and community events

- Work on regional and national projects:
  - Item-writing
  - Review certification exams
  - Work on legislative issues
  - Serve as a regional director
  - Work on an education committee

The Nurses on Boards Coalition (NOBC, 2019) represents national nursing (and other) organizations to build healthier communities through nurses' presence on corporate, health-related, and other boards, panels, and commissions. The NOBC was created in 2014 in response to the Institute of Medicine (2010) report, *The Future of Nursing: Leading Change, Advancing Health*. The report recommended increasing the number of nurse leaders in pivotal decision-making roles on boards and commissions that work to improve the health of the U.S. population.

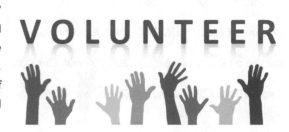

The goal of the NOBC (2019) is to fill at least 10,000 board seats with nurses by 2020. In addition, NOBC seeks to raise awareness about the benefits of having a nurse's perspective in decision-making on issues related to improving health and creating a more efficient and effective healthcare system at local, state, and national levels. For more information about NOBC, visit their website.

Summary

As stated earlier, benefits to joining a professional organization give nurses the opportunity to meet required competencies of a professional registered nurse. Nurses have an opportunity to advocate for themselves the nursing profession (such as the Safe Staffing bill) and serve society by using their knowledge and competencies to improve the health of their communities.

Professional growth and career opportunities are endless. Membership offers many networking opportunities with other healthcare professionals at conferences, involvement in Lobby Days, community events, serving on a board of trustees, and more. Mentoring is a rewarding experience for both the mentor and mentee. By helping nurses gain competencies and confidence, the healthcare system is strengthened, patients receive quality care, which in turn leads to improved patient care experiences and satisfaction rates.

Through organization membership, nurses can fulfill lifelong learning requirements to meet a variety of needs and requirements, such as license and certification renewal and incorporate evidence into practice. Depending on career goals and professional development needs, nurses should evaluate and compare member benefits from different organizations. If a career goal is to obtain specialty certification, it would be prudent to choose an organization that offers reduced fees for a review course. If the goal is to obtain access to evidence-based practice resources for a specialty setting, find a specialty organization that offers these resources.

Since some membership dues can be costly, nurses should check websites for a student discount. Nurses who are unable to join an organization can still benefit from visiting professional organizations websites. Many organizations offer resources to the general public without membership. Echevarria (2018) suggests nurses ask themselves if the organization:

- meets professional growth needs
- aligns with current role/specialty
- meets personal advocacy efforts

Professional organization membership benefits everyone: nurses, the nursing profession, and the entire healthcare system.

References

American Nurses Association. (2015a). *Guide to the code of ethics for nurses with interpretive statements (2nd ed.).* Author.

American Nurses Association. (2015b). *Scope and standards of practice* (3rd ed.). Author.

Echevarria, I. M. (2018). Make connections by joining a professional nursing organization. *Nursing, 48*(12), 35–38. http://doi.org/10.1097/01.NURSE.0000547721.84857.cb

Institute of Medicine. (2010). *The future of nursing: Leading change advancing health.* National Academies Press.

Nurses on Boards Coalition. (2019). *About. Our story.* https://www.nursesonboardscoalition.org/about/

Capitol Beat. (2019, June 19). *The power of Hill day.* https://anacapitolbeat.org/2019/06/19/the-power-of-hill-day/

Printed in the USA
CPSIA information can be obtained
at www.ICGtesting.com
LVHW080028100823
754784LV00009B/591